RECEIVED

JUL 2 3 2008

FREMONT LIBRARY

NO LONGER PROPERTY OF
SEATTLE PUBLIC LIBRARY

SEATTLE

BELMONT LIBRARY

NO LONGER PROPERTY OF
SEATTLE PUBLIC LIBRARY

THE JUICE FASTING BIBLE

THE JUICE FASTING BIBLE

DISCOVER THE POWER OF ALL-JUICE DIETS TO RESTORE GOOD HEALTH, LOSE WEIGHT AND INCREASE VITALITY

SANDRA CABOT, M.D.

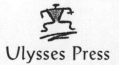

Ulysses Press

Text Copyright © 2007 Sandra Cabot. Design Copyright © 2007 Ulysses Press and its licensors. All rights reserved under International and Pan-American Copyright Conventions, including the right to reproduce this book or portions thereof in any form whatsoever, except for use by a reviewer in connection with a review.

Published by: Ulysses Press
P.O. Box 3440
Berkeley, CA 94703
www.ulyssespress.com

ISBN10: 1-56975-593-0
ISBN13: 978-1-56975-593-8
Library of Congress Control Number: 2007933417

Printed in the United States by Bang Printing

10 9 8 7 6 5 4 3 2 1

Acquisitions Editor: Nicholas Denton-Brown
Managing Editor: Claire Chun
Editor: Mark Woodworth
Editorial and production staff: Amy Hough, Lisa Kester, Tamara Kowalski, Elyce Petker
Cover design: Double R Design
Cover photo: © Liv Friis-Larsen/iStockphoto

Dr. Cabot may be contacted at P.O. Box 5070, Glendale, AZ 85312; (tel) 623-334-3232. Visit her websites www.liverdoctor.com and www.weightcontroldoctor.com.

Distributed by Publishers Group West

NOTE TO READERS
This book has been written and published strictly for informational and educational purposes only. It is not intended to serve as medical advice or to be any form of medical treatment. You should always consult your physician before altering or changing any aspect of your medical treatment and/or undertaking a diet regimen, including the juice-fasting diet as described in this book. Do not stop or change any prescription medications without the guidance and advice of your physician. Any use of the information in this book is made on the reader's good judgment after consulting with his or her physician and is the reader's sole responsibility. This book is not intended to diagnose or treat any medical condition and is not a substitute for a physician.

This book is dedicated to the passionate and knowledgeable group of people who work with me in my head office in Phoenix, Arizona. They are true professionals, always ready to talk to our clients who seek advice regarding their health. They have been with me for many years, and without their help I could not spread the message of the amazing power of nutritional medicine.

Contents

1

Benefits of a Juice Fast

Really, is there anyone who doesn't love a glass of freshly squeezed juice? Or, if you think "love" is too strong a word, perhaps "enjoy" is more your style? Either way, we could be talking about any kind of juice—orange or apple, grapefruit or mango, pineapple or tomato. It's a matter of personal taste and preference, since the list is quite extensive…and becomes even more so if you count vegetable juices as well. But we'll get to that in a while.

For now, let's just relish the thought of what it means to drink a glass of our favorite juice. In my case, it's usually a combination of several juices, which I often rotate from day to day, for variety. First off, juice is flavorful—that's its very essence. Few things please the tongue more. A glass of juice also refreshes us, in a way that colas or one of the many trendy energy drinks could never be. Is it possible that our bodies—unlike our minds—aren't fooled by mega-million-dollar ad campaigns?

Fresh juices are also bursting with all kinds of healthy ingredients: antioxidant vitamins, natural antibiotics, enough beneficial nutrients to stock a health-food store, and anti-inflammatory substances that protect your body's cells as well as reduce pain. Juices even contain enzymes that can improve your digestion and cure some intestinal diseases.

So, if something tastes good and is good for you—and it's also easy to obtain and usually quite affordable—can you think of any good reason *not* to drink plenty of juice? I doubt that you can. But, as you may have gathered from the title of this book, we actually are talking about more here than merely drinking an occasional glass of juice. Rather, we're talking about living for a period of days, or even weeks, on nothing but raw, fresh juice.

Now, while the idea of drinking juice—even a lot of it—appeals to most people, the idea of fasting, even with juices, may not. I'd say that "love" is a word few people would ever associate with fasting, and for the vast majority of us I would imagine that the same holds true for "enjoy." Fasting, as far as most people are concerned, conjures up less-than-pleasant images, such as deprivation, exhaustion, cravings, and a gnawing hunger inside. That sort of feeling, frankly, is quite understandable—with much of the blame falling squarely in the lap of the media, which tell us (or, more often, don't tell us!) the truth about fasting's benefits.

Trace Fasting to Its Natural Roots

By definition, fasting is the voluntary abstinence from solid foods over any length of time. It's a practice that dates back to at least the early days of Christianity and other religions, when it was seen as a way for a believer to purify the soul and prepare to receive atonement for sins. That belief and practice still exists today in some religions. But over the centuries fasting has also been adopted by a wide range of people in an even wider range of cultures, as a desirable way to cleanse the body, calm the soul, and heal the mind. Fasting can be a wonderful thing, as long as it's done properly and not abused.

These days, the only time you will read about fasting in the press, or see it featured in a television news report, might be when a political figure or a political prisoner (self-proclaimed or otherwise) wants to make a statement by starving himself or herself to death, or at least near-death. I believe that this is one of the reasons that many people have a negative image of fasting in general, without really knowing much about it.

A general lack of acceptance by the mainstream medical community has likewise damaged fasting's reputation. This ignorance (for what else can you call it?) has always puzzled me, because many of these same doctors have used fasting's basic concepts to create an often-evil cousin: dieting. If done properly, fasting always works. As for the overall success rate of dieting...well, you be the judge.

Ordinarily, contemporary dieticians and newspaper and television journalists have been conventionally trained to the standards of the day, and have not been exposed to the clinical practice of nutritional medicine to the same depth and breadth as I have been. So it comes as no surprise that many of the fasting articles or detoxing stories we might read in the popular press these days are negative, condescending, sensationalistic, or cynical. Well, let me tell you, the health-care providers mentioned in those stories have usually not treated patients as sick as those I've helped, nor have they witnessed the power of juice fasting as I have done.

It's true that a deep-seated fear of hunger turns many people off to the possibility of fasting, as well as to its benefits. It's a sad fact that in today's world, large numbers of people have serious food addictions. The evidence is all around us, from food-industry advertisements, to the waiting rooms of doctor's offices, to the long lines and even drive-through lanes at fast-food restaurants. It's a hard fact, but a true one, that few addicts would willingly part with their drug of choice, which in this case is poor-quality food.

My hope, however, is that after you read this book and learn the truth about juice fasting and its extraordinary benefits, then you will become as convinced as I am that *there is no better way to improve your overall health*—and your quality of life. Part of the beauty of what you are about to discover is that you can begin your journey to better health doing something as simple, and as delicious, as drinking a glass of your favorite juice.

Avoid Digging Your Own Grave

Whoever came up with the old saying that "You are what you eat" was definitely on to something. This makes it all the more tragic that the vast majority of people in the United States and other developed nations ignore this powerful bit of folk wisdom. And that tragedy has been compounded over the past generation or so, as more and more scientific evidence has shown that many of the most common, and potentially fatal, diseases are directly related to our eating habits.

I suggest a better paraphrase: "You are what you eat…and what you eat just might kill you." I also like the expression,

"The way many people eat today, they're digging their own grave with their teeth."

The average American's diet features absurdly large amounts of refined and processed foods, heavy with trans fats and sugar and practically oozing chemical additives and preservatives. Most commercially raised meats—beef, chicken, and pork—also contain a smorgasbord of additives, which range from growth hormones to antibiotics. And as if this weren't enough to send your body and its elimination systems into overload, imagine the added effect of excess alcohol, caffeine, and nicotine (including secondhand smoke), not to mention polluted air. Then, let's not forget all the pesticides and herbicides and other chemicals that are sprayed on most of our orchards and fields and vineyards, to say nothing about all the plastics that are ubiquitous in our lives. Our waterways become filled with chemicals from plastics, dyes, and even drugs prescribed for people that get improperly flushed down the toilet or are eliminated in their urine.

The Environmental Health Laboratory at the federal Centers for Disease Control and Prevention (or "CDC," for short) conducts the most extensive assessments ever done on the exposure of the general U.S. population to environmental chemicals. It publishes the results every two years in its *National Report on Human Exposure to Environment Chemicals,* which the CDC claims to be the world's leading document on general population exposure. What you'll read in these reports is nothing short of horrifying.

The *Third National Report on Human Exposure to Environmental Chemicals,* the most recent edition, updated the published results from the previous report, in which samples from the 2,000 people tested turned up measurable levels of lead, mercury, cadmium, and other metals; dioxins; PCBs; pesticides; herbicides…the list goes on and on. In total, the *Third Report* updated previous exposure information on 148 different chemicals and included first-time information about another 38 chemicals. That's no fewer than 186 potentially harmful chemicals that were discovered lurking within the bodies of average Americans—that would be you and your family (but not me, as I'm an Australian!).

As I analyzed this information and tried to absorb the enormity of the problem, I could only surmise that it's truly a testament to the strength of the human constitution that most of us in the industrialized Western world manage to live even to adulthood, much less to a ripe old age.

Understand the Body's System for Eliminating Toxins

So, if the food that we eat, the water that we drink, and the air that we breathe are all contaminated (to certain extents) with *toxins,* how do our bodies deal with all these poisons and still survive?

From the day we are born to the moment of our death, our bodies are processing all that we eat, drink, and breathe—

DODGE THE POISONED ARROW

"Toxic" derives from the Latin word for "poison" as well as the Greek word for "arrow poison." The noun "toxin" is derived from that ancient adjective and is included in the International Scientific Vocabulary. Toxins are poisonous substances produced by a living organism's metabolic activity; they must be broken down or excreted before they can build up to dangerous levels. So, whenever we think about toxins arising in our body, we might get a little boost to make some changes in our lifestyle—maybe by imagining poison-tipped arrows being shot directly into our cells.

---

turning some of these substances into useful and beneficial compounds that help us stay healthy, while at the same time filtering, transforming, and eliminating toxic substances and waste products. It's a full-time job, with no days off, and these days a lot of overtime is required.

I think we all agree that ridding our bodies of poisons and toxins would be a good thing, and would certainly be beneficial to both our short-term and our long-term well-being. In a healthy person, the human body is genetically programmed for self-detoxification, so to speak, with the skin, liver, kidneys, intestines, and lymphatic system leading the way. The lungs, colon, and gallbladder provide additional help. In other words, our bodies were designed to naturally eliminate anything they consider toxic.

Liver

The chief engineer of the detoxification process is our liver. It performs hundreds of functions, such as breaking down various toxins into less-harmful byproducts. To simplify what is actually an extremely complicated process, the liver changes fat-soluble toxins into water-soluble byproducts so they can then be eliminated from the body via watery fluids such as bile, sweat, and urine. If your liver does not do this, these toxins remain trapped in the fatty parts of your body—for example, your adipose tissue (that is, connective tissue that stores fat) and your endocrine glands. Little wonder that many people who have become overloaded with toxins have a stubborn weight problem!

Large Intestine

The large intestine, which consists of the cecum, colon, and rectum, is also of major importance. In essence, it is the body's sewer line. Under normal circumstances it functions effortlessly, forming feces and then channeling it out of the body. But, as with a real sewer line, if the large intestine gets overloaded and burdened with excess waste and too many toxins, then it's prone to backing up or malfunctioning. This often means that toxins on the way to being eliminated in the feces are instead reabsorbed back to the poor, overworked liver. If that happens, the detox process becomes like a dog chasing its tail—it does not achieve much at all, except a state of poor health.

Kidneys

A primary function of the kidneys is filtering the blood and removing waste, including many of the toxins that are broken down by the liver and turned into less-harmful byproducts. These byproducts are then eliminated from the body through the urine. In addition, the kidneys maintain the correct balance of such minerals as potassium and sodium in the blood. Drinking a lot of fresh juice and at least 48 ounces of water (6 full 8-ounce glasses) a day are the best ways to keep your kidneys healthy and working properly.

Skin and Lymphatic System

Also helping to eliminate toxins are the skin and lymphatic system. Sweating is one of the obvious ways in which the skin contributes to expelling these undesirable substances from the body. Lymphatic vessels, which drain waste products from body tissue, transport toxins being carried in the lymph fluid to the lymph nodes. In those nodes (also known as lymph glands) foreign particles, including bacteria and cellular debris, are destroyed.

Again, these explanations of how the body's primary elimination systems work are all quite simplified—but there's a reason for that. You need to have a basic understanding of these processes, true. But the real key to this discussion is not how these systems work, but whether they are able, without some help, to do an adequate job of ridding the body of all its harmful toxins. There are two schools of thought on this subject.

In the first school of thought, a number of physicians, scientists, and other experts believe that the body is perfectly capable of handling detoxification on its own. They say that if you are genuinely worried about the negative health effects of toxins, then you should simply change your lifestyle. The focus of this line of thought is diet, because it's generally agreed that up to 80 percent of the toxins in our bodies come from the foods we eat. If you change your diet (or, as one nutrition counselor said, if you "eat closer to nature"), then your body should be able to do just fine on its own. That's one school of thought, and in my mind what it proposes might work very well indeed—*if* we still lived in the Middle Ages!

The other school of thought—the one I personally support—says that modern-day living exposes us to far too many chemicals and other synthetic substances than the average body, or even a healthy one, can adequately handle. As a result, many of these toxins are stored (most often in fat cells) and continue to build up and accumulate until the toxin "dam" begins to crack, so to speak, leaking poisons into the bloodstream and sending them coursing through the body. Also, because we are living longer than our parents and earlier generations, time alone can lead to a more-extensive accumulation of toxins.

Common sense, as well as good science, tells me that we must take whatever steps we can to help our bodies dispose of all these excess toxins. But why, you might ask, does it matter if we lug them around in our tissues and organs?

It matters because an excess of toxins can cause everything from skin rashes, headaches, liver disease, chronic fatigue, and weight gain to much more serious illnesses, such as multiple sclerosis and cancer (to name only two). In fact, though scientific studies have not yet provided evidence to back this up, one expert in the field has said that "all diseases, regardless of their names," are "only varied expressions of the one disease of toxemia" (meaning blood poisoning by toxins that the body's own cells produce). This is a bit of an over-statement, and is too simplistic, since we know that genetic problems are a common cause of disease. Still, my own years of experience with many clients and my own research leave no doubt in my mind that at its core the statement contains more than a kernel of truth.

It all boils down to this: *We must get rid of the toxins that are building up in our bodies, otherwise those toxins—probably sooner, rather than later—may very well get rid of us.* The good news is that the best method of toxin removal starts with—you guessed it!—fasting.

Find Out What a Fast Really Is

Seek out a dozen or so people with personal knowledge of fasting and ask them to define it, and you will likely get a half-dozen different answers. To certain purists, the only true fast is one in which you abstain from all food and drink, with the exception of pure water. A devout Muslim would define fasting as neither eating nor drinking from dawn to sunset every day during the holy month of Ramadan. I myself believe that while juice fasting may not be a "true" fast, it is the best of all options because of the all-around benefits you will receive.

Let me quote Paavo Airola, Ph.D. and N.D. (doctor of naturopathic medicine), who is a well-known believer in juice fasting, who says it as well as anyone ever has done:

> The proponents of the water fast like to tell you that the juice fast is not a fast, it is a liquid diet. They misunderstand the

therapeutic meaning of fasting. Any condition when your body is encouraged to initiate the process of autolysis, or self-digestion, is fasting.

During juice fasting, when no solid foods, proteins or fats are consumed, your body will decompose and burn all the diseased and inferior protein and fat tissues, just as it does during the water fast.

The only difference between the juice fast and the water fast is that during the juice fast your body's eliminative and detoxifying capacity is increased; the healing processes are speeded up and you feel less debilitated. But if someone insists on calling this superior method a juice diet, instead of a juice fast, let him do it if it makes him happy.

To this I would add that if you feel the need to fast—no matter the length of time, which is something we'll discuss in a later chapter—then 99 times out of 100 the underlying reason relates to your desire to improve your health. This can include losing weight. Doesn't it make sense, then, to fast *not* with water alone, but with the raw juices that will provide all the essential vitamins and minerals that your detoxification system needs to eliminate poisons? It has even been pointed out that, for many people, raw juice fasting supplies more nutrients than they were getting in their day-to-day diet.

LOSING WEIGHT BY GOING "CLEAN"

A patient came to see me complaining of excess weight, a rash on her face, and elevated liver enzymes. She had once suffered from acne, for which another doctor had prescribed an antibiotic (tetracycline) for quite a long time. The drug damaged her liver and turned the skin on her face purple. To overcome these drug-induced side effects, she was put on cortisone and antihistamines—which then caused severe heart palpitations.

Eventually, she stopped taking all her drugs and came to consult with me. I started her on a course of juices for her liver and immune system. Within three months, all her problems had disappeared—and she had also lost much of her excess weight.

Boost Your Health by Ingesting Vital Substances

The benefits of juice fasting are a veritable "what's what" of good health. Juices heal and protect your body. They give new life to cells and organs, strengthen your immune system, provide additional energy, help you lose weight, prevent or reverse disease (or both), and even help you look younger and more radiant.

A juice fast, as opposed to a water-only fast, is extremely good at helping an ailing body heal itself. The best available evidence indicates that the minerals and other nutrients contained in juices help break down and dispose of old and dying cells, rejuvenate active cells, and speed up the process of building young and vital cells. Aging and dying cells are one of the primary causes of many different types of disease. Raw juices also contain the following:

- Living enzymes to improve digestion and break down mucous
- Powerful antibiotic substances to fight infections
- Anti-inflammatory substances to reduce pain and swelling
- Antioxidants such as vitamin C, vitamin E, flavonoids, beta carotene, and other carotenoids, which help fight cancer
- Polyphenols are the plant molecules that give color to fruits and vegetables—indeed, all these beautiful and varied colors are even more powerful in their protective and healing effects than vitamins are (the precious polyphenols, which are potent antioxidants, are made much more concentrated by juicing)
- Organic sulfur compounds, which can detoxify poisonous chemicals and cleanse the liver and bloodstream

- Minerals such as magnesium, potassium, calcium, phosphorus, iron, copper, zinc, boron, and selenium
- Vitamin K (found in dark-green leafy vegetables), which is beneficial for bone strength, the immune system, and the blood

Finally, fresh juices contain phytochemicals, substances that can help fight off many diseases. Categories of these chemical compounds include (take a big breath before you read this list!): flavonoids, carotenoids, terpenes, coumarins, capsaicin, chlorophyll, indoles, isothiocyanates, lentinan, and isoflavones. Most of these substances are little known—and certainly a bit hard to pronounce—though they can have a huge impact on your health. Inside one citrus fruit—say, like an orange— are at least 170 phytochemicals that collectively provide anti-inflammatory and antitumor actions, as well as reduce any tendency to form blood clots and offer strong antioxidant activity. In all, more than 4,000 different flavonoids have been identified in the lab, and juicing is the most effective and most economical way to ingest these vital substances in their living form.

It's important to note, too, that juices enable you to take in and use highly concentrated amounts of these phytochemicals, amounts that would be almost impossible to obtain by eating a normal daily-quantity of raw fruits and vegetables.

Trust That Juice Fasting Works

At this point, it would be nice if I could provide a few pages of statistics, or perhaps the results from several accredited scientific studies, to prove beyond any doubt the many benefits of fasting—juice fasting, in particular. Unfortunately, such studies have been few and far between over the years, and so far as I know those that do exist have ignored the benefits of fasting with juices and instead focused on how water-only fasting might be effective in treating specific medical conditions.

For instance, a collaborative study that involved Cornell University found that a medically supervised water-only fast was effective in treating high blood pressure. This is great news; don't get me wrong about that. But because this study appears to be among the more prominent of a limited number of medically supported fasting studies, it also effectively points out that the mainstream medical, scientific, and pharmaceutical communities are almost totally ignoring the full slate of health benefits that can be achieved by fasting, juice and otherwise.

I'm sure I know the reason for this, though it's by no means a good reason: *There's little or no money to be made from fasting.* Invent a new pill that effectively removes toxins from the body, patent it, and market it, and you will make millions, if not billions. Yet sponsor a study that proves the multiple benefits of juice fasting, and all you'll get in return is gratitude and recognition. (Apparently, gratitude has little commercial value.)

Since there is such scant scientific evidence to support juice fasting, I have little choice here but to use a mix of common sense and dietary facts to back my total belief in the value of raw juices and their healing properties.

Stay Away from Poor Food Choices

If you accept the fact—as I do—that up to 80 percent of the toxins entering our bodies come from the foods we eat, then it's pretty much a no-brainer that not eating those foods for a period of time not only will eliminate a major source of toxins, it will also give our toxin-fighting organs a chance to cleanse themselves. To use a homely example, if the drain in your sink occasionally backs up, you don't keep turning on the faucet to add more water. Instead, you use a drain cleaner or a "plumber's helper" tool to clean the pipes. For the human body, raw juices make an excellent drain cleaner.

Fasting also eliminates many problem foods from our diets, at least temporarily. By "problem foods," I mean those containing too much sugar, too much fat, too much salt...well, too much of *many* things that are just plain harmful to our health.

Take sugar, for instance. (Yes, "Please take it away!"—to paraphrase comedian Rodney Dangerfield's old line, "Take my wife...please!") The typical American eats or drinks the equivalent of more than 20 teaspoons of sugar *each day*, according to the U.S. Department of Agriculture, which recommends a maximum of only 12 teaspoons a day (note the word "maximum"). Even 12 is a number that is far too easy to reach. Say that you skip breakfast, then have a 12-ounce cola with lunch, as many of us do. That's 8 teaspoons of sugar right there. Then, midafternoon, you eat a half-cup of canned fruit in syrup—another 4 teaspoons of sugar or the equivalent. At this point, you have reached your maximum daily amount of sugar. Yet for most people, this is only a start to their daily sugar intake.

When you do a juice fast, and thereby eliminate refined sugar from your diet, you not only are saying to your body, "Hey, let's get healthy together!" you are in fact going to actually do that, especially if you have a problem with weight.

Juice fasting helps lower your cholesterol levels, too. Now, to repeat myself, there have been no studies that show this statement to be conclusively based on scientific fact, but how could it not be true? If you don't eat the fatty and/or processed

---

GAIN BY LOSING

Most people who go on a raw juice fast will lose approximately one pound of weight per day. Yes, you read that right: *You can lose one pound each and every day.* Good-bye, baggy figure— hello, slim and trim! Drink up . . .

---

foods that contain saturated fats (which can increase your risk of heart disease and certain cancers) or trans fats (nutritional troublemakers that can increase your LDL, or "bad," cholesterol levels), then there must be some positive benefits, even if your juice fast lasts only for a weekend. And again, two days (or more) without fat entering your system are two days (or more) during which your liver can play catch-up or take a brief rest.

Use Juice Fasting's Healing Power

We live in a world where computers diagnose diseases and, in many instances, play a major role in performing surgery. So, in a sense, it's understandable that many people might tend to minimize natural therapies. Some folks might find it hard to believe that the simple act of drinking fresh raw juices could prevent, or possibly even reverse, serious diseases, while also helping their body rejuvenate itself. Yet I have personally seen juices contribute to improved health in cases in which modern medicine was useless. I have known raw fasts to cure serious diseases in many of my patients suffering such diseases as the following:

- Kidney disease
- Autoimmune disease
- Liver disease
- Cancers of the bowel, prostate gland, blood, and skin

Right now, as you're reading these lines, literally millions of sick people around the globe are searching for lasting solutions to their health problems. In many instances, they're finding that the cure might be as bad as the disease, or even worse. As examples, nonsteroidal anti-inflammatory drugs can damage the stomach, kidneys, and liver when taken over a long period. The cholesterol-lowering drugs known as statins can cause muscle diseases. Some of the drugs used to lower blood sugar levels can cause kidney diseases.

Granted, some people should not undertake a juice fast, and in a later chapter we'll cover the reasons why. But have you ever known a glass of fresh raw juice to cause a medical problem? Neither have I...except for a few, extremely rare cases in which an allergy (sometimes undiagnosed) was involved.

Modern-day medicine often focuses more attention on treating the symptoms of disease, usually with suppressive drugs, than determining the underlying cause. Well, I know for a fact that in many cases that cause is the buildup of toxins in the body—toxins that overload your elimination systems and create health problems that are truly preventable and curable.

I think it's time that we all take a new look, with open eyes, at the treasure-house of nutritional healing methods, so that we can rejuvenate our bodies and bring them back to health, as well as reduce the likelihood of future disease. Even though at the moment you might think a juice fast would be

---

FLY HIGH TO GET GROUNDED IN HEALTH

A friend of mine, a flying instructor, was taking anti-inflammatory drugs to reduce the pain of a back problem. After several weeks, he found himself becoming depressed and unable to remember the things he needed to know to safely fly and instruct students. As he was about to start taking antidepressants, I advised against that and told him to drop the anti-inflammatory drugs and try my liver-cleansing diet and raw juices. He did so, and within two weeks his memory and mental abilities had returned to normal.

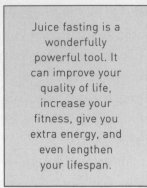

Juice fasting is a wonderfully powerful tool. It can improve your quality of life, increase your fitness, give you extra energy, and even lengthen your lifespan.

too simplistic to do any real good in improving your own health, let me assure you that nothing could be farther from the truth. I hope to convince you otherwise during the course of this book.

I know that I can convince you of the above statement. But before we move on in the next chapter to the subjects of detoxing and "going organic," I want to leave you with three important thoughts:

1. Juice fasting involves *much* more than drinking a few glasses of juice every day.

2. Like every good book or music composition, each juice fast has a beginning that tantalizes you, a middle that engages and informs you, and an end that satisfies you and wraps everything up. (We'll soon cover all three stages in detail.)

3. If you decide you want to fast with juices, do it right and gain all the benefits…or don't do it at all.

2

Detoxing for Greater Health

Over thousands of years civilizations arose, agriculture blossomed in importance and was developed and refined, travel grew from pack animals to supersonic airplanes and even space shuttles, and science and medicine became the bulwarks for a supposedly healthier population. Yet the human body has remained essentially unchanged. How your own body and its internal organs function today is almost exactly how the bodies of your grandparents functioned two generations ago, as well as their own grandparents' bodies and organs two generations before that, and so on and so, on all the way back to the dawn of time.

Considering its complexity and the number of different systems that must function with amazing synchronization, it's obvious to me, and probably to you too, that the design of a healthy human body is about as close to perfection as anything ever gets. I can see only one real flaw (if that's the word for it): that our bodies today haven't changed with the times. They haven't kept pace with the many advances (and in this instance I use "advances" loosely) that have marked civilization's continuing, and often self-destructive, march forward.

Throughout recorded history and up until as recently as several hundred years ago, our environment—the air we breathe, the water we drink, the soil that nourishes the food we eat—was relatively free of contaminants, other than those created by nature as crucial links in the chain of life. What we breathed, drank, and ate was, in almost every case, exactly what our bodies were designed to handle. The necessary nutrients were absorbed, waste products were eliminated, and for the most part our bodies were in balance with both themselves and the natural world.

But jump forward to the 21st century and you'll find that the situation for the vast majority of people living in developed countries has turned by 180 degrees.

At the most fundamental level, maintaining a healthy body seems fairly straightforward: Give it what it needs, stay away from what it doesn't need, and then go about your life as your various organs and systems do their job. What could be simpler? Not much…that is, under ideal or even normal circumstances. Unfortunately, neither exist today. Today's world, in terms of the widespread overabundance of chemicals and contaminants, is the most unnatural environment in the history of humankind. And nothing I have heard or seen or learned of in my medical practice comes close to convincing me that it won't get far worse still.

As recently as the middle of the last century, most of the thousands of manufactured chemicals to which we are now exposed didn't exist. And dozens more are introduced regularly. Our planet—our very home!—is starting to resemble a gigantic dumping ground for garbage and toxins, a chemical stew of unhealthy substances that consistently invade our bodies. When they do, the results are unpleasant at best, disastrous at worst.

It's no coincidence that in the United States, and also in most other developed counties, cancer rates have grown quite high and are rising, while degenerative diseases are major killers. The incidence of obesity and type 2 diabetes has tripled in the past 40 years, primarily because what we are ingesting is not in tune with our bodies' natural needs. Millions of people suffer with liver and gall bladder diseases that are the direct result of a poor diet and a poisoned environment. It's as simple as it is obvious: Good health is difficult, if not impossible, to achieve when your body is burdened with toxins, unhealthy foods, and chemicals.

As a medical doctor, and as a long-time practitioner of holistic healing, I know beyond any doubt that one secret to good health is making sure that your body is properly eliminating toxins and other deadly wastes. While it is doing that hard work for you, *you* should be doing your best to keep new toxins from entering your body, since our bodies' capacity to use nutrients—and to heal itself when sick—is hampered when we allow toxic chemicals to build up.

Cleaning your body of unhealthy materials, and doing it naturally with juice fasting, can and does lead to renewed health and vitality, both physical and mental.

Decide If You Need to Detoxify

If I'm at a social gathering where a friend or family member brings up the subject of the best way to get rid of toxins ("detoxification"), invariably they will ask me two questions: *Do I need to detoxify my body?* and *How can I tell when I do?*

EXTENDING A PRECIOUS LIFE BY RAW JUICES

If my grandmother Susannah Dalton were alive today, she would be at the head of the line of many people willing to testify to life-improving—and, yes, even life-saving—qualities of raw fruit and vegetable juices.

While still in her 20s, my grandmother was stricken with a severe form of a kidney disease called glomerulonephritis. Her immune system attacked the kidneys and caused widespread inflammation, as well as the loss of blood and protein in the urine. In her case, the disease led to severe and life-threatening kidney failure. This was back in the 1930s, when doctors, and medical science in general, offered few, if any, treatments for this type of disease.

The available doctors of the day told my grandfather, Harry Dalton, that they could do nothing further to help Susannah, who at that point was hospitalized and at death's door. Fortunately, Grandfather Harry was a dietician and a man truly ahead of his time. He took my grandmother home from the hospital and started her on a program of drinking raw juices. Every hour on the hour, he gave her a glass of raw juice, which he made alternately from produce that grew below ground (root vegetables) and produce growing above ground.

Over six weeks, my grandmother gradually regained her health, as the kidney inflammation settled down and her kidneys resumed their normal function. In effect, the concentrated minerals, vitamins, and antioxidants in the juices calmed her immune system and put out the fire of acute inflammation. Grandmother Susannah, a thoroughly wonderful woman, was given an extra half-century of life by the power of raw juices. She lived that time to the fullest, before passing away at the then-ripe old age of 78.

I could answer the first question broadly, by telling them since they live in the Western world (that is, not in Asian countries) and eat what's considered to be a "normal" diet— one containing refined sugars, processed fats and grains, preservatives, and fruits and vegetables that at some point have been sprayed with pesticides—then the answer is "Yes." I believe that virtually every reader of this book could benefit from an occasional raw juice fast. To answer the second question for you, the reader, below I have listed a number of easy-to-identify signs and symptoms that may crop up whenever a body laden with toxins is crying out for a thorough cleansing.

I tell my friends and my clients that I firmly believe a juice fast can improve their health and well-being, and possibly can add quality years to your life. I can't offer concrete scientific evidence to back up this claim, since there have been no formal juice fasting studies of any substance—at least, of which I'm aware. But I have been convinced by the amazing positive results I have seen in my own patients, and also among my family and friends, over my 30 years spent practicing clinical medicine.

In my medical practice I have seen raw juices reverse cases of cancer, inflammatory bowel disease, autoimmune diseases, sinus infections, asthma, chronic fatigue, and other illnesses.

Determine Your "Body Toxic Score"

To find out whether your body is overloaded with toxins and could therefore benefit by detoxifying, calculate your personal "body toxic score." Read the list of symptoms below. Mark 1 point next to each symptom that you have at least once a month.

___ Bad breath
___ Coated tongue
___ Skin rashes and skin infections
___ Excessive weight that just won't shed, despite dieting
___ Itchy skin
___ Overheating of the body
___ Excess sweating
___ Brown liver spots on the skin
___ Cellulite

___ Swollen glands

___ Dark circles under the eyes

___ Headaches that are recurrent

___ Digestive problems—nausea, reflux, stomach ulcers

___ Red, itchy eyes

___ Body odor

___ Strong odor to the urine

___ Offensive flatulence

___ Constipation

___ Irritable bowel syndrome

___ Inflammatory bowel disease

___ Recurrent infections

___ Severe allergies

___ Hormonal imbalances

SCORING YOUR NEED FOR A DETOX

2 points	You *could* benefit from a juice fast
3–6 points	You *should* consider a juice fast, sooner rather than later
7 points or higher	A juice fast is just the thing to improve your health and well-being, and could add quality years to your life

I'm confident that very few of you reading this have not experienced a half-dozen or more of these symptoms, at least occasionally. That means that very few of you—perhaps none—will derive no benefit at all from a juice fast.

But before I go any further, to cover subjects that range from picking out your fruits and vegetables and beginning a fast, to what to do during a juice fast and how to come off one safely, I'd like to touch on how juice fasting can truly help people suffering from one of the world's most common and physically damaging medical conditions: excess weight.

Think of Juice Fasting as Nature's Fat Burner

I'm sure that the weight-reducing potential of doing a juice fast will interest may of you great, since one-third to one-half of all adults living in developed countries are fighting a daily battle with their weight…and, more often than not, they are losing. Want proof? Just glance around you at people in your office or walking down your street, or take a look at ordinary people shown on your evening news program on television.

A lot of these people—I'd say the vast majority—think they're overweight because they eat too much or too often, or perhaps don't exercise enough, or have inherited the wrong genes from their parents. Indeed, all these circumstances can lead to a weight problem. But at the same time, blaming excess body fat on any or all of these three causes is often too simplistic and far too limited. Any number of medical problems, including fatty liver and body toxicity, can be responsible for many of those extra pounds.

If you recall, in the first chapter I explained how the chief engineer of the detoxification process is the liver, which performs hundreds of functions, including breaking down a variety of toxins into byproducts that are less harmful. The liver changes fat-soluble toxins into water-soluble byproducts; these can then be eliminated from the body by bile, sweat, and urine (being watery fluids).

If the liver fails to do this, the toxins stay put, trapped in fatty body parts like adipose tissue and endocrine glands. *Many people who struggle with keeping their weight down are, in fact, overloaded with toxins.*

An unhealthy liver is also less effective in removing small fat-globules that circulate in the bloodstream. This will cause excessive fat to build up gradually in various parts of the body, including other organs, as well as in fatty deposits under the skin. Many adults who bear excess fat in the upper part of their abdominal area have, in fact, what doctors term a "fatty liver." The liver has stopped burning fats (thus getting them out of the body) and instead has become a fat-storing organ. If you yourself have a fatty or enlarged liver, like a goose being force fed to make foie gras (literally, "fatty liver"), you will not be able to lose weight, regardless of what diets you might try, until you first improve your liver function.

Also, if you overload your liver with too many medications, such as antibiotics, strong hormone-replacement therapy drugs, or cholesterol-lowering drugs, your liver's biochemical pathways will have fewer remaining energy reserves to perform that organ's normal duties of metabolizing fats. This, too, can be a cause of weight gain. A fatty liver tends to accumulate fat-soluble toxins, which further slow its ability to burn fat.

Yet once you start a raw juice fast, your liver will immediately recognize that the almost-nonstop stream of toxins and fats that it was previously processing has subsided. Your liver will react to this change by shifting into an entirely new mode

---

BATTLING A FATTY LIVER

One of my patients suffered from longstanding obesity. She had tried stomach stapling, fad diets (some of which possibly were dangerous to her health), and seemingly tons of appetite-suppressant drugs. The latter had damaged her liver and she had developed what doctors call a "fatty liver," which made it impossible for her to lose weight.

I convinced her to start juicing and to take a liver tonic. After 12 months, she had reversed her fatty liver and lost more than 75 pounds. Fresh juices, she had discovered, quenched her appetite and gave her the energy to start exercising, which further helped her health gains.

of operation: releasing its own stored-up fats and toxins, while also drawing in fats and toxins from other parts of your body and processing them for elimination, too. Your liver then becomes the powerful, fat-burning organ it was meant to be, and it can do its other job of pumping unwanted fats and toxins out of your body via the bile.

So, as you can see, just giving your liver the gift of better health will—by itself!—cause a lot of those unwanted pounds to melt away. When you add the fact that someone on a juice fast is significantly reducing his or her intake of both calories and fats, then it's as plain as the glaze on a donut why a juice fast can, and often does, lead to weight loss of up to one pound each day—with the people who weigh the most generally losing the most.

And, unlike many diets, a juice fast—as I mentioned in Chapter 1—is healthy, because your body is receiving an increased measure of all the vitamins, minerals, and antioxidants that it needs. In fact, a juice fast, if done properly, will give you the essential nutrients that your body requires to clean and repair its cells while also strengthening your immune system.

Choose the Best Fruits and Vegetables

Like so many other things in life, not all fruits and vegetables are created equal. You will definitely want to keep this in mind when selecting your produce.

Why? Well, first and foremost, you know by now that one of the primary reasons to go on a juice fast is to rid your body of unwanted and unhealthy toxins. Therefore, you will be far better served if you eat organic produce instead of produce that has been sprayed with pesticides and herbicides and all

---

TO 'CIDE OR NOT TO 'CIDE?

When you hear words like "pesticide" or "herbicide," do yourself a favor and think of their origins. The "-cide" compound is borrowed from Latin terms for "cutter," "killer," and "slayer"—giving us such unfortunately familiar words as "homicide," "suicide," and "infanticide." An insecticide, for instance, destroys the bugs bedeviling your flowers, an herbicide kills the crabgrass in your lawn...but what do other "-cides" do to *you and yours* when you eat their residue on your fruits and vegetables?

---

the other "-cides." Yet these chemicals, sad to say, contaminate most of the produce that's commercially available today, including what is sold at almost every corner market, at every large supermarket, and at many farmers markets as well.

Go Organic

Organically grown produce should *always* be your first choice, but unfortunately that choice may not always be available. Growing fruits and vegetables organically is always time- and labor-intensive, which makes it costly and the direct opposite of everything that most large commercial growers believe in. Their main interest is in profit, not quality—and certainly not in improving my health or yours.

If you can't find organic fruits and vegetables in your corner of the world, or at all seasons of the year, then at least make sure that you always wash them well in running water (not a basin of standing water) and (if appropriate) peel them before juicing. This will eliminate most harmful chemicals.

If you're not completely sure whether your peelable fruits and vegetables are genuinely "organic"—fruits such as nectarines, apricots, apples, beets, carrots, and all citrus varieties—just peel them, as added insurance. Remember that canned or frozen fruits and veggies, as well as once-fresh varieties that have been stored for long periods or gas ripened, are not suitable for juicing. Whenever possible, choose produce that is fresh and in season (at least, in season somewhere in the world, wherever it's flown in from!).

In this same vein, if you happen to be strolling through a park or woodlands, do not—I repeat, *do not*—pick plants to take home for juicing. Dandelions are a good (well, a bad) example; many people find that dandelion-leaf juice makes a tasty and healthy addition to a number of juice combinations. And while it's true that its leaves are high in vitamin and mineral content, if you pick leaves at random you may also be getting a concentrated pollutants from animals, industry, automobiles, and various lawn and garden fertilizers and herbicides. In other words, you could easily be getting more bad toxins than good nutrients, thus defeating your purpose.

READ "ORGANIC" LABELS WITH A SPOONFUL OF CAUTION

Wherever you buy your produce (whether at a farmer's market in a public square, in a health-food store, or in a supermarket), be a bit cautious. If you see the word "organic" used on a sign or pricing label, know that it may have been used either correctly (to your benefit) or loosely (perhaps to your harm).

"Organic vegetables," depending on whose definition you believe, have been treated (if at all) with fertilizers or pesticides of strictly animal or vegetable origin.

"Organic chicken," if accurately labeled, has been raised without the use of drugs, hormones, or synthetic chemicals.

I advise you to interpret other uses of "organic" as loosely descriptive ("Come dine in our all-organic restaurant!") or sometimes as out-and-out flimflam (as when marketers claim that "Our products will ensure you a simple, healthful, and close-to-nature organic lifestyle").

Buyer beware!

Another major drawback to indiscriminately picking leaves and plants is the plaintive cry of a sick person: "But it looked like the real thing!" Many plants in nature have a "copy"—a fraternal twin, so to speak—that not only looks enough alike to be confusing but may also be poisonous, or at least foul tasting. As you progress in your juicing regimens, if you develop a taste for plants found mostly in nature, you can grow them organically in a small garden or a large pot on a porch or deck, or you can search out (through friends, or perhaps online) a specialist nursery nearby that grows them in a controlled situation.

Finding a plant in nature is no guarantee that it, in fact, is "natural." Maybe that particular plant was, once upon a time, but realistically it isn't today.

Find Your Own Favorite Combinations

When deciding which fruits and vegetables to juice, and in what proportions or combination, remember that some of the recipes you'll find in Chapter 7 are only general guidelines. Feel free to experiment with new things, and change ingredients to suit your taste and the season.

Through (dare I say bitter?) trial and error, I have found several combinations of produce that do not mix well in

---

FOLLOW DOCTOR'S ORDERS, PLEASE
I recommend that you not change the proportion of fruits to vegetables in my suggested recipes; otherwise, you may take in too much sugar. At first, as with anything new, the results of your experiments might not always be to your liking—but don't be discouraged. The very next combination you try could absolutely work magic on your taste buds! This has happened to me more than once.

---

juices. This can result in a combination that tastes unpleasant or maybe doesn't sit well on your own digestive system. From experience, I have learned that you'd be wise to avoid the following combinations:

- Prune juice does not go well with cabbage, onion, watercress, or garlic
- Pear juice and tomato juice are not a good mix
- Grape juice combined with carrot juice can cause flatulence (gas)
- Garlic and onion juice do not taste good with fruit juice (except tomato, lemon, and orange juices)
- Fig juice mixes poorly with radish juice
- Blackberry juice does not get along with beetroot or its leaves
- Apricot juice does not do much when combined with green vegetables or green leaves
- Cabbage, watercress, or turnip juice does not mix well with lemon or grapefruit juice

If you find that a particular combination of juices does not make you *and* your mouth happy, then you have three choices:

- Strike these juices off your list.
- Alter the balance, until it suits your taste.
- Dilute the juices with water to see if this makes the drink more palatable.

If you haven't already realized this, then you'll soon discover that when you're juicing things and then tasting the combinations, the terms "healthy," "beneficial," and "tastes good" won't always spring to mind! Juice combos can literally be an acquired taste. But I promise you that I've come to love the taste of certain raw juice combinations that previously would have struck me as tasting peculiar.

Follow These Juicing Principles

It's true that some juices are a bit hard to take in their pure form. And, as with many other things, personal preference will always come into play when selecting the produce you'll juice. As I say that, however, I would also add that regardless of the likes and dislikes of your taste buds, knowing the following facts will help every juicer:

- Choose produce that is as fresh, unblemished, and in season as you can get it.

- Wash all produce well, removing any bruised, blemished, or moldy parts. Cut or slice the produce into pieces to fit into the input of your juice extractor.

- The white inner skin (pith) of citrus fruits is full of beneficial bioflavonoids, so try to always include some of this when juicing these fruits.

- Most bottled juices are nearly worthless in terms of fasting, having been pasteurized for shelf longevity—a process that destroys enzymes and many vitamins.

- Before juicing fruits containing large pits, such as peaches, pit them, to keep from tearing up your juicer.

- Include in your juices the stems and leaves of vegetables (except carrot tops, which can cause kidney stones), because they have a high vitamin and mineral content.

- Do not wash green vegetables in hot water for a long time, or leave them to soak in cold water, as this draws out many beneficial minerals.

- It's best to drink juice within one hour of making it; otherwise, if left out on a counter it can be oxidized by exposure to air and may develop a sour taste.

- If you must make juice ahead of time, store it in a jar with a tight lid or in the refrigerator in a closed container.

- When making virtually any juices, you can add a bit of lemon juice to preserve the natural color and help reduce the oxidation of essential nutrients.
- If you have irritable bowel syndrome or an otherwise sensitive stomach, make sure that you dilute your juices with water (*rule of thumb:* 3 parts juice to 1 part water). People with this condition often tolerate celery juice when mixed with fruit juices.
- If losing weight is your primary concern, use mainly vegetable juices, since they contain fewer calories than do fruit juices.
- Some fruits (cantaloupe, for instance) are highly pulpy and contain little juice; some berries (such as blackberries and blueberries) contain relatively little juice and may be unsuitable for juicing.
- Dried fruits such as raisins or apricots obviously contain no juice, though you can soak them in water for half a day and then drink the water to enjoy their flavors and nutrients.
- Always wash your produce under the tap, because even organic fruits and vegetables can carry bacteria and parasites. The tap water will carry the bacteria and parasites down the drain.
- If you are pressed for time, make several pints of juice at a time, then freeze them in daily serving-size containers. The juice must be frozen immediately after making it and must be drunk immediately after thawing.

After you have read the next few chapters, and as you begin your own experiments with juicing, you'll likely discover other properties and combinations—so share these with your friends, family, and fellow juice-fasters. In my own case, this happens to me all the time! As with all journeys, your discoveries and successes (both large and small) along the path to better health will add to your pleasure when you reach your goal.

3

Best Fruits and Vegetables for Juicing

Throughout the previous two chapters, I've frequently mentioned both *fruit* and *vegetable* juices as being good for your health. Yet, with the exception of juice from the tomato (which is actually a fruit) and a popular commercial product that contains the juices of several vegetables, most people think of "fruit" when they hear the word "juice." That's true of many of my patients, as well. Even at my seminars, when those attending know they will hear about all kinds of juices, people seem shocked to learn that in a proper raw-juice fast most of the juice should come from…wait for it…raw vegetables.

One of the fun things about juicing is that once you get into the rhythm of it and start trying various juice "recipes," you'll discover that you are going to love the many juicing options you'll find in the wide world of vegetables. And not only will their juices make you healthier by helping to clear toxins from your body, and particularly from your liver, in many cases (also just like fruit juices) they are extremely tasty, too. Fantastically so!

First-time juice fasters often ask me whether taking in nothing but juices—be they fruit, vegetable, or a combination of the two—might not be too much of a good thing. My answer is always the same: *Absolutely not!* In fact, not only do juices soothe your digestive system, they also come packed with living enzymes to assist in digestion. Giving your intestines, liver, and pancreas a little break by an all-juice diet will be a nice vacation for them, as they can easily extract from the juices all the vital nutrients your body requires. And after drinking juices you will never feel heavy or weighted down, as you often do after a full "normal" meal.

When you fast with juices, you absorb up to 99 percent of their nutritional value. They provide a concentrated supply of vital nutrients, especially antioxidants. Drinking a medium-sized glass of carrot juice (8 ounces), for example, is the equivalent of eating a little more than 1 pound of raw carrots. You can imagine that eating that many carrots at one sitting would take a good deal of time and would also be fairly hard on the teeth and jaws. Few things are more enjoyable, however, than drinking an 8-ounce glass of fresh, tasty carrot juice.

It's worth noting here, too, that the vast majority of fruits and vegetables offer benefits that go well beyond improving

---

"AUNTY WHO?"

Antioxidants are substances that may protect cells from the damage caused by unstable molecules known as free radicals. They do this by interacting with and stabilizing free radicals, and in the process may prevent some of the damage that free radicals otherwise might cause. Examples of antioxidants include beta carotene, lycopene, and vitamins C, E, and A.

---

the health of the body's elimination systems. Apples, for instance, are beneficial for massaging the gums, reducing gouty arthritis, and lowering cholesterol—and, besides that, they taste great and come in myriad varieties (especially if you can find a farmers' market, or buy your apples direct from the grower at a roadside stand). Beetroots can reduce hardening of the arteries, red radish can fight infections, and turnip leaves can strengthen bones, nails, teeth, and hair. And this is only a small sample of the overall health benefits that are derived from the regular consumption of fresh juices.

The bottom line (and many of you who are worried about your weight will be watching your "bottom" line) is that you really can't go wrong when you include both fresh vegetable and fresh fruit juices in your diet. This is true whether you're fasting, or simply enjoying a daily glass or two of juice with your meals, or looking for a healthy pick-me-up between meals. Below is a list of many of my favorite vegetables and fruits, that breaks down the vitamins and minerals and other good things that each contains, and briefly sums up how each can help your body heal and strengthen itself as it waves "Good-bye! And don't come again!" to years of accumulated toxins and unwanted fat.

Know Your Fruits and Vegetables: Produce Vitamins and Minerals Benefits

ALFALFA SPROUTS
Vitamins: B, C, E, K, folic acid, and beta carotene.
Minerals: magnesium, sulfur, chlorine, silicon, calcium, iron, zinc, sodium, potassium, and phosphorous.

Benefits: Supports liver function and assists with weight loss. Helps to balance the hormones.

APPLE

Vitamins: B and C.

Minerals: potassium, calcium, phosphorous, iron, silicon, and chlorine.

Benefits: High in the soluble fiber pectin, which soothes the intestines and heals stomach ulcers. Improves colonic flora and reduces unfriendly colonic bacteria and parasites. Aids in digestion. When juiced, the core, skin, and flesh increase mineral and antioxidant content.

APRICOT

Vitamins: B, C, and beta carotene.

Minerals: sodium, calcium, potassium, iron, magnesium, and phosphorous.

Benefits: Excellent for skin problems. Helpful in cases of inflammatory bowel disease.

ASPARAGUS

Vitamins: B, C, folic acid, and beta carotene.

Minerals: calcium, iron, phosphorus, potassium, and magnesium.

Benefits: Its juice helps to protect the kidneys, as well as reduce the likelihood of kidney stones.

BANANA

Vitamins: B and C.

Minerals: calcium, magnesium, and potassium.

Benefits: Excellent for stomach and intestinal inflammation. Green (unripe) bananas can heal certain cases of inflammatory bowel disease, such as ulcerative colitis.

BEAN SPROUTS
Vitamins: B, C, E, and beta carotene.
Minerals: calcium, iron, and potassium.
Benefits: Cleanse and detoxify the entire body.

BEANS, STRING
Vitamins: B, C, beta carotene, and folic acid.
Minerals: calcium, iron, magnesium, and potassium.
Benefits: Used by practitioners of Oriental medicine to strengthen the liver and kidneys. Reduce blood sugar and insulin levels, and thus aid fat burning. Great for diabetics.

BEETROOT AND TOPS
Vitamins: C, B, folic acid, and beta carotene.
Minerals: chlorine, manganese, calcium, iron, phosphorous, potassium, chromium, and magnesium.
Benefits: Good cleansers for the liver and biliary system, which transports the bile made in the liver (which pumps out toxins via the bile into the gut for elimination).

BLACKBERRIES
Vitamins: B, C, and beta carotene.
Minerals: calcium, iron, and potassium.
Benefits: Blood and skin cleanser. Helpful for intestinal inflammation. Reduces Alzheimer's dementia.

BLUEBERRIES
Vitamins: B, C, and beta carotene.
Minerals: calcium and potassium.
Benefits: Useful in cases of intestinal inflammation and skin problems, as well as a good blood cleanser. Reduces Alzheimer's dementia.

BROCCOLI
Vitamins: B, C, folic acid, and beta carotene.

Minerals: calcium, iron, phosphorous, magnesium, potassium, and sulfur.
Benefits: Excellent for weight loss. Helpful for sluggish liver function.

BRUSSELS SPROUTS
Vitamins: B, C, folic acid, and beta carotene.
Minerals: phosphorous, calcium, iron, magnesium, potassium, and sulfur.Good general tonic.
Benefits: Helpful for liver problems and obesity.

CABBAGE
Vitamins: C, B, folic acid, and beta carotene.
Minerals: very high in sulfur and chlorine; also contains magnesium, calcium, potassium, and iodine.
Benefits: Excellent for many digestive and intestinal problems. Excellent liver tonic. Reduces disorders of the bile ducts. Good skin cleanser.

CANTALOUPE
Vitamins: B, C, and beta carotene.
Minerals: calcium and potassium.
Benefits: Useful for kidney problems.

CARROTS
Vitamins: B, C, D, E, K, and beta carotene.
Minerals: calcium, iron, phosphorous, chromium, potassium, iodine, silica, chlorine, and sulfur.
Benefits: Excellent for skin problems. Reduce inflammation of the mucous membranes in the intestines. Are a liver cleanser and tonic. Superb for increasing vitality and vigor. Improve eyesight, especially night vision.

CAULIFLOWER
Vitamins: B, C, folic acid, and beta carotene.

Minerals: calcium, iron, phosphorous, magnesium, sulfur, and potassium.
Benefits: Excellent liver tonic. Useful for kidney disorders.

CELERY
Vitamins: B and C.
Minerals: calcium, iron, phosphorous, potassium, magnesium, sodium, iron, and sulfur.
Benefits: Reduces acidity, which is beneficial when trying to overcome toxicity. Excellent for stomach problems such as ulcers and reflux. Reduces fluid retention. Reduces arthritis. Excellent for weight reduction, as it lessens a "sweet-tooth."
Note: Cut pieces into short lengths so that long fibers won't become twisted in the juicer.

CHERRIES
Vitamins: B, C, and beta carotene.
Minerals: phosphorous, potassium, and iron. Darker cherries contain greater amounts of magnesium, iron, and silicon.
Benefits: Good blood cleanser.
Note: Are extra-beneficial for juice fasters who might suffer from anemia, rheumatism, asthma, or high blood pressure.

CHIVES
Vitamins: B and C.
Minerals: selenium, phosphorous, iron, chromium, calcium, sulfur, magnesium, and potassium.
Benefits: Contain allicin, which fights infection and reduces LDL ("bad") cholesterol. A good liver and bile cleanser. Natural antibiotic for the whole body. Dispel intestinal parasites.

CITRUS FRUITS (see also Grapefruit and Oranges)
Vitamins: Very high in C. Also, the white pith on the inside of the skin contains large amounts of valuable flavonoids.

Minerals: potassium, magnesium, sodium, calcium, and phosphorous.

Benefits: Contain natural antibiotic, anti-inflammatory, and cleansing properties. Are powerful antioxidants. Soothe inflamed mucous membranes. Reduce the risk of heart disease, blood clots, and strokes. Improve eyesight.

COCONUT MILK

Vitamins: B, C, and E.

Minerals: calcium, phosphorous, potassium, and iron. Good source of protein.

Benefits: Serves as an excellent base for combination juices that contain other fruits. Contains natural antibiotic substances.

CORIANDER LEAVES

Vitamins: B, C, and folic acid.

Minerals: potassium, sodium, and magnesium. The active ingredient in coriander is volatile oil.

Benefits: Stimulate the flow of bile and relieve stomach and intestinal cramps. Fresh coriander helps with indigestion. Improve liver detoxification.

CRANBERRY

Vitamins: B, C, and beta carotene.

Minerals: sodium, potassium, copper, calcium, manganese, phosphorous, iron, zinc, magnesium, and sulfur.

Benefits: An excellent skin cleanser and tonic. Prevents urinary tract infections.

CUCUMBER

Vitamins: B, C, and beta carotene.

Minerals: sodium, silica, manganese, sulfur, potassium, calcium, phosphorous, chlorine, and magnesium.

Benefits: Reduces acidity and soothes the stomach, intestines, and urinary tract. Its rich silica content is beneficial for skin and hair. Enzyme content aids protein digestion. Reduces kidney stones and arthritis.

DANDELION
Vitamins: high levels of beta carotene, folic acid, and B, with good levels of C.
Minerals: high in potassium, calcium, iron, and magnesium.
Benefits: Cleanses the liver and biliary system. Stimulates the flow of bile and is useful in all liver complaints. Also a blood builder, helpful for anemia. Juice is extracted from the leaves of the plant, which must be used fresh and washed thoroughly.

FENNEL
Vitamins: B, C, and beta carotene.
Minerals: calcium, chromium, cobalt, iron, magnesium, manganese, phosphorous, potassium, selenium, silicon, sodium, and zinc.
Benefits: Has a calming effect on digestion and stimulates gastric secretions. Reduces intestinal cramps and flatulence.

FIGS
Vitamins: B, E, C, and beta carotene.
Minerals: calcium, iron, phosphorous, magnesium, and potassium.
Benefits: Helpful if you have problems gaining weight. Have the highest sugar content (about 50%) of common fruits, so are best avoided if losing weight is one of your juice fasting objectives. Reduce constipation.

GARLIC CLOVES
Vitamins: B and C.
Minerals: selenium, phosphorous, iron, chromium, calcium, magnesium, and potassium.

Benefits: Contain allicin, which fights infection and reduces LDL ("bad") cholesterol. A good liver and bile cleanser. Natural antibiotic for the whole body. Dispel intestinal parasites. Reduce blood clots and heart disease. Fight respiratory and sinus infections.

GINGER ROOT
Vitamins: C.

Minerals: copper, potassium, sodium, iron, calcium, zinc, phosphorous, and magnesium.

Benefits: Natural antibiotic for the whole body. Reduces mucous production and congestion. Inhibits the formation of blood clots and lowers LDL ("bad") cholesterol. Reduces arthritis and relieves pain.

GRAPES
Vitamins: B, C, and beta carotene.

Minerals: phosphorous, iron, calcium, and potassium.

Benefits: Provide a quick energy boost. Support skin, kidney, and liver function. Help eliminate acid from the body. When juicing, use the whole fruit, including skins. Keep refrigerated.

GRAPEFRUIT
Vitamins: B, E, beta carotene, biotin, and inositol; very high levels of vitamin C.

Minerals: calcium, iron, phosphorous, and potassium.

Benefits: Helpful for obesity, sluggish liver function, and respiratory and skin problems. Reduces blood clots and strokes. Natural antibiotic. If you are taking prescribed medications, tell your doctor if you are using grapefruit regularly, for it can interact with several medications.

GUAVA
Vitamins: B, C, and beta carotene.

Minerals: calcium, iron, potassium, and phosphorus.

Benefits: Helpful with digestion and improves circulation. Reduces blood clots.

HONEYDEW MELON
Vitamins: B, C, and beta carotene.
Minerals: calcium, phosphorous, potassium, and iron.
Benefits: Helps with kidney problems and skin conditions. Aids in weight loss.

HORSERADISH
Vitamins: B and C.
Minerals: phosphorous, calcium, and sulfur; high in potassium.
Benefits: Dissolves mucous. Natural antibiotic, especially good for sinus infections. Stimulates the flow of bile and elimination of toxins via the liver.
Note: Excess amounts can irritate the stomach.

KELP (and also other Sea Vegetables, such as Arame, Wakame, Nori, Hijiki, and Dulse)
Vitamins: B and beta carotene.
Minerals: calcium, magnesium, potassium, iron, phosphorous, iodine, selenium, and zinc.
Benefits: An excellent source of minerals and trace elements that are not readily obtainable in many of the more popular vegetables. These sea vegetables' rich mineral content strengthens the immune system and boosts thyroid function, making them an excellent aid to weight loss in those with a sluggish thyroid. Alginic acid, present in many types of seaweed, binds with heavy metals such as lead, mercury, and cadmium and enhances their elimination from the body.
Note: Avoid kelp and other seaweeds if your thyroid gland is highly overactive (hyperthyroidism).

LEMONS
Vitamins: C and P (from the citrine content).

Minerals: potassium, magnesium, and small amounts of calcium.
Benefits: Excellent cleanser for the liver, bowel, and blood.
Reduce the risk of blood clots, strokes, and heart attacks. Are
a powerful antibiotic.

LETTUCE

Vitamins: B, C, and folic acid.
Minerals: calcium, silica, potassium, phosphorous, sulfur,
iodine, iron, and magnesium.
Benefits: A primary benefit of lettuce to juice fasters is its abil-
ity to calm the nervous system and help improve sleep.
Reduces fluid retention and arthritis.

MANGO

Vitamins: B and C; high in beta carotene.
Minerals: calcium, iron, phosphorous, and magnesium.
Benefits: Helpful for inflammation of the stomach, and
improves digestion. Enhances skin appearance and healing.

NECTARINES

Vitamins: C and beta carotene.
Minerals: calcium, iron, and phosphorous.
Benefits: Support digestive activity. Exert cleansing properties
in the intestines. Reduce constipation.

ORANGES

Vitamins: very high in C. Also, the white pith on the inside of
the skin contains large amounts of valuable flavonoids.
Minerals: potassium, magnesium, sodium, calcium, and phosphorous.
Benefits: Contain natural antibiotic, anti-inflammatory, and
cleansing properties. Powerful antioxidant, and reduces the
risk of blood clots, strokes, and heart attacks. Lower cholesterol. Give quick energy boost. Improve eyesight.

PAPAYA

Vitamins: B; high in C and beta carotene.

Minerals: phosphorous, potassium, iron, and calcium.

Benefits: Contains the digestive enzyme papain (a valuable digestive aid). Cleanses the stomach and intestines. Soothes the stomach and heals intestinal ulcers.

PARSLEY

Vitamins: B and folic acid; high in C.

Minerals: sodium, calcium, magnesium, potassium, phosphorous, copper, and manganese; high in iron and chlorophyll.

Benefits: Excellent cleanser of the liver, kidneys, intestines, and blood. Reduces constipation. Helpful in cases of anemia.

PEACHES

Vitamins: B, C, and beta carotene.

Minerals: potassium, sodium, magnesium, calcium, phosphorous, and iron.

Benefits: Quick energy booster. Improve the skin. Reduce stomach and kidney inflammation. Reduce constipation.

PEARS

Vitamins: B and C.

Minerals: calcium, iron, phosphorous, potassium, sodium, and magnesium.

Benefits: Useful for digestive problems, irritable bowel, constipation, and colitis. Of great benefit in those with food allergies and sensitivities. Provide quick energy boost.

PEPPERS—SWEET

Includes those that are green, red, orange, yellow, and purple (members of the capsicum family)

Vitamins: beta carotene, folic acid, and B; high in C.

Minerals: potassium, silica, iron, calcium, phosphorous, and magnesium.

Benefits: Powerful cleanser of the intestines and liver. High antioxidant content. Powerful antibiotic for the whole body. Reduce risk of blood clots, heart attacks, and strokes. Improve eyesight.

PEPPERS—CHILI

There are more than 200 types of chili peppers that range in taste from mild to blisteringly hot; red chili peppers are not always hotter than the green but are likely riper.

Vitamins: beta carotene, folic acid, and E; very high in C.

Minerals: potassium, magnesium, sodium, and selenium.

Benefits: Chili peppers provide many health-related benefits. Of greatest interest to juice fasters is their effect of increasing the metabolic rate, thus assisting with weight loss. In excess amounts, can irritate the stomach and intestinal lining (use caution if you have digestive or intestinal problems). Reduce blood clots, heart disease, and stroke. Powerful antibiotic to fight infections. Improve eyesight.

PINEAPPLE

Vitamins: B, E, and C.

Minerals: calcium, sodium, phosphorous, potassium, chlorine, and magnesium.

Benefits: Has anti-inflammatory properties. Supports digestion of proteins. Assists in weight reduction.

POTATOES—REGULAR

Vitamins: B and C.

Minerals: iron, potassium, and phosphorous.

Benefits: Soothing to the stomach intestines. Reduce acidity and fluid retention.

Note: there are thousands of varieties (discard potatoes with green patches, as these contain toxins called solanines)

RADISH AND RADISH LEAVES
Vitamins: B, C, folic acid, and beta carotene.
Minerals: calcium, iron, phosphorous, silica, sodium, potassium, magnesium, iodine, and chlorine.
Benefits: Excellent liver and bile cleanser. A natural antibiotic for the entire body. Reduce the levels of LDL ("bad") cholesterol. Reduce blood clots.

RASPBERRIES—RED
Vitamins: B, C, and beta carotene.
Minerals: iron, potassium, and phosphorous.
Benefits: Assist with weight loss. Strengthen the immune system.

RHUBARB
Vitamins: B, C, and beta carotene.
Minerals: calcium, iron, phosphorous, potassium, and sodium.
Benefits: Improves the flow of bile and gastric juices. Helps support the muscular action of the bowels and small intestines. Preferably used in small amounts in mixed juices, as it contains high levels of oxalic acid. Should be avoided if you suffer from arthritis or kidney stones.
Note: Never use the leaves, as they can be toxic.

SPINACH
Vitamins: B, C, K, choline, inositol, folic acid, and beta carotene.
Minerals: iron, calcium, magnesium, phosphorous, potassium, and sulfur.
Benefits: Quick energy boost (remember "Popeye," the sailor man?). Reduces muscle cramps. Lessens heavy, painful menstrual bleeding. Good general cleanser.

STRAWBERRIES
Vitamins: B, C, and beta carotene.
Minerals: potassium, calcium, iron, and phosphorous.

Benefits: Excellent skin cleanser. Reduce constipation. Have antioxidant effects.

SWEET POTATOES

Vitamins: B and C; very high levels of beta carotene.

Minerals: calcium, iron, phosphorous, potassium, silicon, chlorine, and sodium.

Benefits: Have a soothing effect on an inflamed stomach and colon. Improve hormonal balance.

TOMATOES

Vitamins: B, C, K, and beta carotenes, including lycopene, which has anticancer properties.

Minerals: potassium, calcium, iron, phosphorous, and iodine.

Benefits: Good liver and bile cleanser. Antioxidant properties. Reduce prostate problems, such as enlargement and cancer.

TURNIP

Vitamins: B, C, E, and beta carotene.

Minerals: calcium, iron, phosphorous, sulfur, and potassium.

Benefits: Excellent liver and bile cleanser. Best combined with carrot or apple juice, as there is a slightly bitter taste.

TURNIP LEAVES

Vitamins: B, C, E, K, folic acid, and beta carotene.

Minerals: iron, sulfur, phosphorous, and magnesium; high levels of calcium.

Benefits: Good blood and liver cleanser. Help with digestive problems and gall bladder inflammation and gallstones.

WATERCRESS

Vitamins: B, E, C, folic acid, and beta carotene.

Minerals: calcium, iron, sodium, magnesium, phosphorous, chlorine, potassium, and iodine; very high in sulfur.

Benefits: Excellent cleanser for the liver and bile ducts. Supports kidney function and reduces fluid retention. Good skin cleanser. Best when mixed with other juices.

WATERMELON
Vitamins: B, C, and beta carotene.
Minerals: calcium and iron; very high in potassium.
Benefits: Supports kidney function and reduces inflammation in the intestinal tract. Cleansing effect on the skin.

WHEAT GRASS
Vitamins: B, C, E, K, folic, B17 and beta carotene.
Minerals: calcium, zinc, magnesium, potassium, phosphorous, sodium, sulfur, and cobalt. Very high in chlorophyll.
Benefits: Powerful cleanser and detoxifier of the liver and blood. Strengthens the immune system. Has antiaging capabilities.

Experiment, to Suit Your Taste

As you skim the chart, reading details that catch your eye about your favorite fruit or veggie, you likely have noticed that many of those listed are quite similar in their vitamin and mineral content, and many have the same uses as well. This is where your taste buds come into play. If you find that you don't care for a particular combination of juices—say, one that contains a particular vegetable, even though it's a fine liver and blood cleanser—then just replace it with another fruit or vegetable that offers the same benefits. The potential combinations are almost endless. If you experiment, you're almost guaranteed to find the combinations that are right for you.

Enjoy Your Beta Carotene

While we're on the subject of vitamin and mineral content, I'd like to point out that the majority of fruits and vegetable contain beta carotene. This is a powerful antioxidant that can reduce your risk of many types of cancer—ones that often are caused by the toxins in the material we eat, drink, and breathe. If you undertake a juice fast of any length, it's possible that levels of beta carotene will build up in your body. When this happens, a slight yellowing or bronzing of the skin may occur. It will probably be more apparent on pale areas, such as your palms or inner arms. Do not be alarmed. This is nothing to worry about and is entirely harmless. Many people are told that this can lead to vitamin A toxicity, but that is definitely wrong. Your body will make vitamin A out of beta carotene only if the body *needs* more of that vitamin. Indeed, a high level of beta carotene in your body will do nothing more than reduce your risk of cancer, while giving your skin a healthy, tanned look without the dangers often caused by too much exposure to the sun (and without the cost and time of using a tanning booth!).

Choose Your Ideal Juicer

Finally, before I move on to subjects directly related to fasting, it's important that I give you a brief tour at the three most common types of commercial juicing machines—if for no other reason than that you can't begin a juice fast without one. (Juicing by hand is too laborious and simply is not doable.) While I won't recommend any juicers by brand name, I will cover the advantages and disadvantages of each general type of juicer. Then I'll leave it to you to take this information and find a juicer that best suits your personal needs and budget. It may be a good idea to educate yourself by doing some online shopping and comparing models and prices, even reading comments from "happy buyers," but you will probably be more satisfied with your purchase if you visit a store to handle and lift and actually test a machine in person.

Centrifugal Juicer

The centrifugal type of juicer first chops your produce into small pieces and then throws them against a spinning bowl, which separates the fiber from the juice. In my opinion, this type is not as efficient as a masticating juicer, though the more expensive ones will certainly get the job done.

Advantages: • Is easy to clean
• Tends to be relatively inexpensive

Disadvantages: • Can be extremely noisy
• May clog if produce is fed in too fast
• Has a shorter life span
• Does not extract the juice completely, wasting more of the produce

Masticating Juicer

Like a miniature version of a wood chipper, a masticating juicer chews and then grinds the produce into tiny particles. Then it presses or mashes them through a screen, thus separating the juice from the fiber.

Advantages: • Has a somewhat longer life span (being made typically with high-quality parts)
• Is easy to clean
• Can easily juice all grasses, such as wheat grass
• Offered in the medium-priced range

Disadvantages: • Can be heavy and cumbersome (in certain models) to clean and store

Hydraulic Press Juicer

The third type of juicer uses both a hydraulic press *and* a grinder. The pressing action turns fruits and vegetables into a paste, which is then pressed further to extract virtually all the juice. Of all three types of juicers, this one allows the greatest proportion of juice to be separated from the fiber pulp.

Advantages: • Has the longest life span (having been made with high-quality parts)

• Can readily juice grasses, such as wheat grass

• Is the most efficient juicer among the three types

Disadvantages: • Is the most expensive type of juicer

Ready...Set...Start Juicing!

There's not a lot left to say about juicing itself. Once you have tested several juicers (many health-food stores even provide some produce for you to experiment with) and chosen the type that suits you best, you'll find it simplicity itself to extract your juices. The final step: Take your machine home, rinse some fruits and veggies, and try out your new best friend.

I do want to stress one thing, which by now will not surprise you in the slightest: I have no doubt at all about the many health benefits you can—and will—derive from raw juicing. Few, if any, things are better for your physical and mental health. Having said that, and hoping that your own experiences with juicing will soon have you nodding in agreement with me, I'll move on to fasting.

In the next chapter, we'll talk about how a fruit and vegetable juice fast, when done properly, can forever improve your life—and indeed may even save it.

4

Juice Fasting Safety and Preparation

Whenever I talk to patients or friends and family about juicing and fasting, selling them on the idea of drinking a lot of fresh fruit and vegetable juices is the easy part. It's a bit like talking a 6-year-old into eating an ice-cold popsicle on a hot summer's day: nothing to it. But ask that same young boy or girl, on that same hot summer's day, to drink a steaming cup of broccoli soup…well, the look you might get is close to what I sometimes see when I start talking up about the wonders of fasting.

Now, I realize that if I once again stress the benefits of fasting here, I'll largely be preaching to the choir. Most of you wouldn't have bought this book, or wouldn't be reading it, if you didn't already believe—or want to believe—that fasting with fresh, raw juices is a good and healthy thing to do, and that it can improve quality, as well as length, of life by cleansing and rejuvenating the body. Many people find that it helps their soul, as well. But, as I said, that's the belief of *most* of you. Most, but not all.

It was my great fortune to grow up with a mother who constantly read, and who just as constantly passed on to me her favorite books. Most were interesting or educational, or both. Many became my own personal favorites. But some of those books—and specific subjects aren't important—I finished simply because I was expected to. In these cases, my enthusiasm for what I was reading was often less than stirring. Maybe it was because I didn't, or couldn't, buy into the book's message, and therefore took away nothing after having read it. Perhaps I found fault in the author's reasoning. Sometimes these books were plain dull. Worst of all, though, is when they weren't convincing.

As a lover of words and thoughts who spends countless hours reading, and countless more hours writing, I believe that not being convincing is one of the worst sins any nonfiction author can commit. So, dear reader, if you are someone not already singing in the "juice fasting choir," or are reading this book merely because it was recommended to you, or because the passenger before you left it in your taxicab, let me try this one final time to be convincing.

As a juice faster myself, and as a medical doctor who has prescribed and administered juice fasts to countless others, I have found absolutely nothing in either conventional or holistic medicine that can compare to raw juice fasting for ridding an unhealthy body of years of accumulated toxins, and for encouraging your unwanted pounds to melt away like that popsicle on a sizzling summer's day.

If a car analogy works better for you, you can even put fasting in the same category as having your car regularly serviced. Think of it as preventive maintenance, but for your own personal chassis and transmission. Do the maintenance every few thousands miles (or the human equivalent) and you might be surprised how many extra years of good service you'll get out of your aging engine.

So...juice fasting is a good and healthy thing to do. Period. No doubts. And it can improve the quality of your life, as well as the length of it. If you are not convinced, just try it. Then I'm sure you will be.

Be Aware of a Few Yellow Flags

Having said this, my preaching is finished, though I almost feel guilty for now having to point out that, unfortunately, fasting is not for everyone. Speaking as a medical doctor, I realize that a very few people should not fast. Therefore, I'll wave a few yellow flags below; if the cautions do not apply to you, you can proceed right on down the track.

If you are one of the people who shouldn't fast—and you will soon find out whether you are—you can still enjoy the taste and many of the benefits of the juices of fresh fruits and vegetables, only you can't do it as part of a fast. In your case, it would not be the healthy thing to do.

Observe Basic Requirements for a Fast

As far as I'm concerned, both as a doctor and as a faster myself, you only need to note three simple requirements for fasting:

- You should be in relatively good physical health.
- You should be comfortable with yourself and in a good place mentally—not feeling desperate, for instance, to lose weight because you're about to spend a week at the beach.
- You should fast only if it's something *you* want to do, not something that someone else is encouraging you to do.

As with most every human activity, fasting will definitely be more enjoyable—and possibly more effective too—if you approach it with a feeling of excitement about what's to come, rather than looking at it as a chore, a means to an end, or something that needs to be done but gotten over with quickly. I suggest that you view your fast as a trip to a vacation wonderland, not a visit with a cranky relative.

In a later chapter, we'll discuss the various physiological and psychological effects of fasting. For now, let me emphasize once more that fasting needs to be something that you really want to do for yourself—and for the right reasons.

TALK TO YOUR DOCTOR

With these thoughts in mind, I also recommend that you talk with your physician or a health-care provider who is familiar with fasting if you are planning a juice fast that will last more than a day.

Fasting is not advised for quite a few medical and health-related conditions and situations. For example, pregnant or nursing women should never fast. Why? First, a woman's body has other priorities at these times, and babies (whether inside the womb or out) do require regular amounts of protein for proper growth and 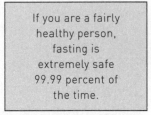 development. Why upset the body's normal routine at a time when it's already under a lot of stress, trying to support the nutritional needs of two people? Also, juice fasting starts a detoxification process that quickly increases the number of toxins circulating within your body, even as they are on their way to being expelled. Common sense, as well as medical science, tells you that a many of these toxins could easily be car-

> If you are a fairly healthy person, fasting is extremely safe 99.99 percent of the time.

ried to a baby, either through blood if the baby is still in the womb, or in breast milk if the mother is nursing. Infusing a newborn with a larger-than-necessary load of toxins is not giving that baby the best possible start in life. So pregnant or nursing moms will simply need to wait awhile to discover the benefits of juice fasting. But better late than never, right?

NOTE OTHER CONDITIONS THAT RULE OUT FASTING

As a rule, certain people should never juice fast, or water fast, or do any other kind of fast. These are people who suffer from any of the following conditions:

- Diabetes
- Low blood sugar
- Heart failure
- Liver failure
- Kidney failure
- Eating disorders, such as bulimia or anorexia nervosa
- Epilepsy
- Low blood pressure
- Moderate to serious asthma
- Gout
- Malnutrition
- Tuberculosis

If you suffer from one or more of these conditions, any change in what your body is used to will add stress (mental and physiological) to your system. And stress is never good when your body is already in a battle for its health or, in extreme cases, fighting for its continued existence. So before you begin a juice fast, it's a good idea to do a little research, use your common sense, and talk to your physician if you have any health concerns.

Although the conditions are the most common among all the medical reasons for not fasting, certain other chronic and acute conditions are also incompatible with extended fasting. Again, it's important to get a professional opinion before you start a juice fast—especially one that will last for more than several days.

A few medical conditions, however, are borderline as regards fasting. Cancer is the leading example. Some medical professionals will tell you *never* to fast if you have cancer, since that disease is essentially an indicator that your immune system is in poor health. Other doctors, including me, hold the belief that since juice fasting is so very nourishing, usually more good than harm will come when a cancer patient undertakes a brief raw juice fast (of, say, two to three days). But let me repeat: Consult with your health-care professional before you commit to a fast.

DO NOT STOP YOUR MEDS WITHOUT A DOCTOR'S APPROVAL

It needs to be mentioned, too, that if you are taking prescribed medications, you should never stop them abruptly—even when fasting—without your doctor's permission and support. It's possible that after fasting for a few days, you may be able to reduce your dosage of some medications because of changes in your body. But never do it on you own, without a doctor's OK. To do so could be a fatal mistake.

Certain medications—such as blood-thinning drugs or anticoagulants, or drugs that must be taken with food—may cause stomach upset or be less effective during a juice fast. Fasting can reduce blood proteins and therefore change the way medications react in your body. If you take prescribed medications, always discuss this topic with a medical professional before you begin a juice fast.

WAIT OUT ROUTINE SICKNESS BEFORE YOU FAST

Nor do you want to begin a fast if you are sick or just getting over an illness, even if the illness is just a cold or a mild case of the flu. In either situation, your immune system is under stress and your body already has enough to cope with. It's wise to wait a few days or a week, until you're feeling normal again, and *then* start your juice fast with a clean slate. And never start a fast right before, or right after, a surgical procedure. Again, the reason is that you should not place too much stress on your body at any one time.

As you'll read in a later chapter, fasting—in spite of its many benefits—does put a certain amount of stress on the body's organs and systems. And they will have to adjust to the different fuel mix you are giving them for a while.

PUT CHILDREN ON A FAST CAUTIOUSLY

There is no good reason to put young children on a fast, except perhaps at times when they are ill and naturally have no appetite. At all other times, a child's rapidly growing brain and body require maximum nutrition. This can change, however, when a child enters the latter stages of his or her teenage years. Then, the wisdom of a juice fast depends on the individual— whether the young person is mature enough to recognize the need for and the benefits of an occasional full-body detoxification. If the child happens to be yours, you will know him or her well enough to know what's right, and what to recommend.

PREPARE FOR YOUR FAST

If you have made it through the last page or two without discovering a medical reason for *not* fasting, now it's time for you to turn your attention to how to prepare for a fast—what to do before you actually begin. As with many things in life, common sense reigns, though I will throw in some professional advice, as well. Let's start this discussion not with you, but with your surroundings.

I assume that by the time you reach this point (not in my book, necessarily, but in your preparations for fasting) you will have already purchased or otherwise obtained a juicer. That's actually a pretty significant step, your first real commitment to a new and healthier lifestyle. Place the juicer in the kitchen, next to your sink. Then, head straight for the pantry, before moving on to your refrigerator, to get rid of those chips you like so well and, oh yes, that container of onion dip. Toss out all the cupcakes, cookies, and pastries. Give that half-gallon of ice cream to the neighbor's kid (no, not the tubby one, but the skinny one who is always willing to help around your yard).

In other words, get rid of all the processed and fat-laden foods that may tempt you during your fast. I'm not implying that you lack willpower, or that you can't resist the siren call of your favorite midnight snack (though I know from experience it can be hard at times). It's just that I see no reason to make a new and enjoyable experience more distracting, or in any way more difficult, than it absolutely needs to be. Common sense, again.

DISCUSS YOUR FAST SPARINGLY WITH OTHERS

For first-time juice fasters especially, please don't discuss your plans with friends or family any more than necessary. I'm not worried about the people who'll try to discourage you—some will!—but I do think that your focus should be on *you* and what you are preparing to accomplish for yourself, rather than what others might say or think.

This is not about ego, or about being the first in your social circle or on your block to try something new. Fasting shouldn't be a fad. Fasting is about improving your health, about feeling good inside and out. As someone wiser than me once said, the only person you need to impress is yourself.

GET GOOD EXERCISE

It's also a good idea to have in mind some sort of exercise plan, if this is not something you currently do. If you don't know much about fitness, the first step for anyone beginning an exercise program—particularly if you are age 35 or older—is to have a thorough exam by your physician or health-care provider. Request that this be done during the visit you'll be making to discuss your juice fasting plans. Next, begin to consider activities that you know you will enjoy. Bear in mind that you won't want to do extremely challenging exercise during a juice fast, because you may be tired then and need extra rest.

Choosing an exercise is very much a matter of personal preference. For some people, it can be as simple as gardening or working in the yard. Others may like to learn a new sport, such as tennis or bowling. Walking and jogging are popular, as are yoga and swimming. It truly doesn't matter what exercise you choose, as long as it's something you enjoy and something you do for at least 30 minutes on most days of the week.

Once you settle on exercise activities, the first rule is to not overdo it. Start by warming up for three to five minutes, followed by three to five minutes of the kind of stretching related to your particular exercise. It's important to stretch, and to do so properly, before *and* after exercise. Most people know about stretching, but don't know how to do it correctly. Each stretch should be held for 20 to 30 seconds and repeated several times. Stretches must never hurt. One caution I give is to *never* do bouncing stretches, as they can and do cause injuries by themselves.

No matter what activity you choose, try to keep a gentle pace that allows you to talk and move comfortably while doing it. I say this because some people tend to go crazy at first and do too much, too fast. If you do overdo it and injure yourself slightly, one of the secrets to quick recovery is RICE (Rest, Ice, Compression, Elevation of the injured limb).

"What's all this about exercise," you might be wondering? "Isn't this a juice fasting book?" Well, yes, it is—but juice fasting and exercise share a common focus: taking better care of yourself and doing something that will make you healthier and also will make you *feel* healthier and hold yourself in higher regard. Besides, I've found that many people who didn't normally exercise, but began a light exercise program as part of their fasting plan, stayed with the exercise afterward. Juice fasting by itself is great; I just can't recall anyone ever saying it needs to be one-dimensional.

SCHEDULE YOUR FAST THOUGHTFULLY

Another consideration here—and some people will deem this more important than others—is the best time of year to fast, particularly if you are a newcomer and intend to fast for more than a day or two at a stretch. Some proponents recommend that fasting be done only during the warmer months of the year, spring being the optimal time. Others say that the season makes no difference and that what's more important are what's going on in your life at a given time and whether fasting will mesh with those other activities. You obviously don't want to plan a juice fast to coincide with a family hiking vacation, the start-up of a new business, or the week you'll be on your honeymoon.

In my opinion, warm-weather months are generally preferable, particularly for all first-time juice fasters. My reasoning is that in a cold environment your body must generate

---

HAVING YOUR JUICE ON THE GO

Ideally, you should drink juice within an hour of making it, otherwise it can be oxidized by the air and may, in some cases, develop a sour taste. If you must go to work or be away from your juicer for most of the day, make several juices in advance and store them correctly. Use a jar with a tight lid or a jug with plastic wrap sealing the top, and keep them cool in a refrigerator if possible.

---

additional energy just to stay warm and comfortable. Having said that, however, I'll fall back on my mantra of common sense and recommend that you look at your life in its entirety, not taking into account only the season or the weather, and then time your fast based on that full picture.

Many people also wonder whether it's OK to juice fast and still go to work or carry on with their normal life activities. For most people and most juice fasts, especially those lasting three days or fewer, my answer is "yes." Circumstances will vary from person to person, but if you are in decent health and have a job that doesn't require extreme physical activity, or if you aren't planning to swim the English Channel or climb Mount Whitney, then just continue with your job and your daily activities. It's not uncommon to feel more energized and productive while fasting. But if you are on a fast, regardless of the length, and you feel a bit weak, it's fine to take a vacation day, or hang around the house instead of hiking with friends. The key is listening to your body and, once more, using common sense. Do both, and it's hard to go wrong.

FOLLOW A PRE-FAST DIET

Now that I have laid the external groundwork for fasting, let's turn our focus in the other direction and look internally. I strongly suggest that a minimum of five to seven days before beginning your juice fast—no matter its planned duration—you remove all animal products from your diet. This includes meat, poultry, fish, eggs, and dairy. Also, cut out all greasy and deep-fried foods. And begin significantly reducing your intake of caffeine, alcohol, nicotine, chocolate, candies, sugar, coffee, and colas.

By the third day before your fast begins, your diet should basically consist of fruits and vegetables, nuts and seeds, and

---

TO SUPPLEMENT OR NOT

People contemplating a juice fast often ask me this: "Should I take vitamin or mineral supplements?" Frankly, I don't recommend either one, for three reasons. First, taking a pill on an empty stomach may cause a little upset. Second, many vitamins and supplements work properly *only* if taken with foods. Third, if your juicing is balanced and includes several varieties of both fruits and vegetables, you should be getting all the vitamins and minerals you'll need.

---

beans. Any stimulants should be history by now, a distant memory. Then, on the day before you start fasting, eat nothing but uncooked fruits and vegetables—preferably organic, if these are available.

This gradual (but total) removal of cooked and processed foods in the days leading up to a fast is based on a medical fact: To go overnight from your normal diet and lifestyle to a diet and lifestyle consisting only of raw juices can cause your body to detox *too quickly,* making you feel uncomfortable at best, or slightly ill at worst.

PREPARE YOUR MIND AND SPIRIT, TOO

Getting yourself ready both mentally and emotionally is also important, and something I strongly recommend to anyone fasting for the first time. Give careful thought to what it is you'll be doing and what you hope to accomplish. Walk your mind through the benefits of fasting. Mentally consolidate your reserves of willpower, so that you'll be ready to react in a positive way when a forgotten candy bar suddenly leaps out of a drawer and straight into your hand ("positive way" means that you immediately put it back or toss it into the garbage!). Realize that you may experience some emotional ups and downs when you begin to fast—but know that, as with most things, these feelings will soon pass.

What will also pass are the feelings of hunger that almost everyone feels on Days 1 and 2, and sometimes even Day 3, of a longer fast. I assure you that such hunger almost always goes away by the end of Day 3, and from then on most people will find that the longer they fast, the less hungry they'll feel. Notice that I said "most people," because everyone will react a bit differently. There is no real reason for concern if you don't feel hungry and it's just Day 2, nor should you be concerned if you are still hungry on Day 4.

In all respects—not just in regard to fasting—you are an individual, and as such your body is going to do what it needs to do. "Go with the flow," as white-water river runners say, and don't let hunger issues put a damper on your fasting experience or your longer-term goal. Hunger doesn't deserve a second thought during a short fast or in the initial days of a longer one. Any hunger you feel during the final stages of a longer fast is simply your body telling you that perhaps it's time to break the fast (more on this later).

FAST SAFELY AND USE COMMON SENSE

Finally, you need to be aware of the need for safety. A fast is supposed to help you, not hurt you. And it won't hurt you if you properly prepare for it, follow the guidelines in this book, and take to heart any conditions or restrictions that your physician or other health-care provider recommends. Do all these things, and your fasting will be as safe and comfortable as if you were a child again curling up in your loving mother's arms.

Safe fasting begins with the correct preparation, which has been covered in this chapter. It continues through the fast itself (see Chapters 5 and 6), and ends when you come off the fast and resume a normal diet (Chapter 8).

Again, as much as than anything else, fasting safety is about using your God-given common sense. Think about it: Do you recall a time when you looked well, even felt well, but somehow knew that you were about to come down with the cold, or that by the next day you'd probably start to feel flu symptoms? Have you ever had a feeling that something wasn't quite right with your body, and even though you couldn't pinpoint the problem you went to see you're your doctor anyway—only to learn that you were indeed sick? I see patients all the time who come in for these or similar reasons. To me, this is a perfect example of common sense at work, medical style.

What I mean by that is, if something doesn't feel right—if your instincts are telling you, "Hey, pay attention, because we've got a problem here"—then you should listen and act on it. I'm a big believer in following your instincts.

Yes, your body will start to experience a lot of changes, both physical and mental, as you begin to fast. And, yes, toxins that have been lying dormant in your body for years will be stirred up and agitated by the fasting process, and will probably even wreak a little internal havoc as they begin their forced exodus. This internal activity, along with a total lack of the solid food you're so used to, may make you feel things you've never felt before. And while some of these feelings may be good, others likely won't be so pleasant.

Regardless, I'm convinced that if you pay close attention to your body and what it's telling you, you'll be able to differentiate between the normal internal feelings that come with fasting and the abnormal feelings that indicate something isn't going as it should.

I'm not trying to scare you here, because I am totally convinced that if you are a fairly healthy person, *fasting is extremely safe 99.99 percent of the time.* I only mention the possibility of that other, minuscule 0.01 percent, because I'm a medical doctor and I'm sworn to always protect the health and safety of my patients. And while those of you reading this book are technically not my patients, I tend to see you that way and feel that you deserve the same consideration.

Use common sense, listen to your body, follow your instincts, take corrective action if necessary (such as breaking your fast or seeing your doctor)—and finish reading this book. Then I assure you that your juice fasting will be as safe as it will be beneficial.

5

Choose a Program
for Your Fast

We've now arrived at a point where you are comfortable with
the idea of juice fasting and excited about its many potential
benefits, physical as well as mental. I'd be the first to admit
that I'm excited *for* you, as you are about to have a positive,
life-altering experience that could forever change your perspective on a number of health- related topics, from eating
habits to weight control. If you've never fasted, you might
think I'm a bit nuts to say this. But I even hold the opinion
that successfully completing a first fast can be one of life's
most rewarding moments. It may even be comparable to
receiving a long-sought promotion at work, or hearing that
you have been named your community's leading citizen.

If for some reason, however, you are still not "comfortable" with or "excited" about the prospects of a juice fast, then
I recommend that you step back and reassess your motivation
for considering a fast. As I've said before, in so many words,
and as I'll continue to say throughout this book, if the timing
isn't right, or if your heart isn't into beginning a fast, then your

body certainly won't be into completing one. You must be ready if you hope to realize the maximum benefits.

Think About How Long You Want to Fast

For those of you who are prepared to move and to begin your fast, the obvious question you're asking yourself will be: *How long should I fast?* The answer is another question: *Is this your first fast?*

If it is your first time, —and it probably is for most of you, then shorter is initially better than longer. Compare it to jogging. If you decided to take up jogging as a way to relieve stress or drop a few unwanted pounds, you wouldn't go out on the first day in brand-new running shoes and enter a five-hour marathon, or even a 10K race (that's 6.2 miles, for those who don't speak "metric"!). Or, I should say, you wouldn't do so if you have any sense at all.

No, instead you'd break in your equipment, then on your first day you'd warm up, then jog around the block or through a neighborhood park, then cool down and rest. You would refrain from entering a long-distance race until after your body had adjusted to jogging. You would want to gain both experience and know-how—as well as good all-around "body awareness"—*before* you entered a long race, to avoid causing yourself more harm than good. The same principles can be applied to fasting.

Start off slow, get your feet under you (so to speak), and if you find that you are enjoying the experience and the benefits of a short jog (or fast), then build on that and add to it with longer runs (fasts)...until you reach your ultimate goal of a 10K race (a seven-day fast) or even a marathon (a prolonged fast of two weeks or longer). The important thing is, if you try to do too much, too soon, you'll likely have a less than pleasant time of it and will end up retiring your running shoes (your juicer) to the back of the closet, where they (it) will never again see the light of day.

Start Cautiously, if You're a First-Timer

If you happen to be doing any research on fasting beyond this book—particularly if you are doing Internet searches on the topic—you will likely come across information that says it is perfectly OK for virtually everyone to fast for 14 days or longer. And it *is* OK...just *not* for everyone. If you have fasted before and you know first-hand the physiological and psychological effects (see Chapter 6) that often accompany an extended fast, and if you feel that this is the right time in your life and it is something you really want to do, then go for it. And enjoy it all the way.

But if you're a first-time faster, I'd recommend that you ignore this information. In fact, put it out of your mind. Don't listen to these people.

I could be polite here and say that everyone is entitled to an opinion, and that any "expert" who suggests that 14 days is a suitable length for a first fast may know something that I don't. When it comes to your health, however, honesty is more important than politeness, so instead let me say the following.

I'm a licensed medical doctor, I graduated from a top medical school, and I have spent more than three decades practicing conventional medicine. Over that same time span I have also studied and practiced holistic medicine. Based on this accumulated knowledge, it is my professional opinion that anyone who says it is OK for a first-time faster to consider a fast of longer than two days is wrong. Dead wrong (well, not literally "dead"). And I'm about to explain why.

First, however, I'd like to digress for just one paragraph to point out that, along with the 1-day fast, this chapter will cover the reasons for and benefits of a 2-day fast, a 3-day fast, a 7-day fast, and fasts of 14 days or longer—all done while drinking raw fruit and vegetable juices, of course. We'll also touch on some other beneficial practices that go hand-in-hand with fasting, such as colonics and enemas, dry brush massages, and steam baths. But, back to the 1-day fast…

Do a One-Day Fast

Anyone who is in decent physical condition, has a good mental attitude, and is not very young or very old can easily and safely undertake a one-day fast, despite having no fasting experience whatsoever. I think you might be surprised at the many positive things that can come from something as simple as replacing your normal diet (which, for most of us, is not all that great) with fresh fruit and vegetable juices…for only 24 hours. (In Chapter 7, you'll find a lot of great recipes for doing exactly that!)

To many of you, it may seem that going without food for 24 hours is a really high hurdle, especially if you are used to eating two or three big meals a day, along with one, two, three, or even more in-between-meal snacks. But trust me, it's not that difficult!

For starters, if you begin your fast in the evening of Day 1, after dinner (and that would be a dinner consisting of uncooked fruits and vegetables, not steak and fried potatoes), then bedtime will follow shortly, and by the time you wake up the next morning your fast will already be halfway over. At that point, you will just have to go without food for 10 to 12 hours, until dinner on the evening of Day 2—but again, it will be fruits and vegetables, with perhaps some beans or a few nuts, not pizza and beer.

Watch What You Eat, Before and After

I have to be honest here and admit that the meals leading up to a one-day fast, as well as those that immediately follow, don't necessarily have to be as free of fats and sugars and spices and carbohydrates as they would if you were undertaking a much longer fast. In truth, some experienced fasters will argue that part of the beauty of a one-day fast is that is

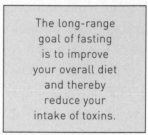

The long-range goal of fasting is to improve your overall diet and thereby reduce your intake of toxins.

doesn't require much, if any, preparation on the front end, or any change in your normal routine after the fact.

Though I'm not able to disagree with this point of view from either a medical or a health-related standpoint (at least not too strongly), I do find it an exceedingly narrow view. For it fails to take into account what I believe is a primary long-range goal of fasting. That goal is to improve your overall diet and thereby reduce your intake of toxins.

I don't disagree that a one-day fast, even if it's squeezed in between meals of steak and pizza, can still do a lot of good. But I do question how much more good might result if the before-and-after meals were a little healthier, and a bit more conducive to fasting. You'll have to be the ultimate judge on this one, at least as far as your own fast is concerned. But I know what *I'll* do: I will continue to eat the healthiest available foods, both right before and right after I fast, regardless of how long the fast.

Of course, it goes without saying (so I'll say it) that we all should be eating those "healthiest available foods" all the time. We aren't, of course, or at least the vast majority of us aren't. But that's a story for another day.

As you are already aware, every human being is different in some respects, and everyone will react somewhat differently to fasting. So it's hard to say specifically how you, being a unique individual in the universe, will benefit from a one-day fast. In general terms, however, a 24-hour diet of nothing but raw fruit and vegetable juices will give your body a chance to rest some of its systems and focus for a time on cleaning and repair.

If you've every worked in a large office or in a high-rise building, then you're probably familiar with the cleaning crews that come in at night, when all but the most necessary work has ceased, to collect the trash, vacuum the floors, and otherwise get the office or the building ready for the next workday. It's the same with fasting.

On a one-day fast (or on a longer fast, for that matter), your body can temporarily forget about digesting food and storing toxins, and instead it can concentrate on cleansing itself and getting rid of chemicals and replacing damaged or diseased tissue. During a fast, energy that would normally be used for processing food is used instead for repair.

Get a Good Start on Your Detoxing

Now, I'm not about to claim that fasting for a single day can turn your health around or cure an illness or get rid of an ailment. But many, many people will bear me out on the fact that a one-day fast can, and does, give you a fine start on detoxing your body. If you follow up with additional one-day fasts or go to longer fasts, then the improvements in your health will certainly come much faster and will definitely be more noticeable. It's like the people on that cleaning crew—if they neglect to mop and wax the kitchen floors for a few years, or a few decades, then the first mopping won't make much of a difference. But with each successive mopping, the floors will get cleaner and cleaner, and, with a little persistence they'll be shining like new.

A one-day fast has still another benefit: to teach you to control your cravings and desires for unhealthy food. For most of us, a significant proportion of what we eat is not really doing us much good, aside from keeping us alive. In many cases, it is actually doing a great deal of harm. Yet we tend to continue waltzing down the same dietary path until our blood pressure shoots sky high, or our cholesterol starts climbing, or our heart protests all the ill-treatment by having an attack—or sometimes until we start avoiding mirrors because we no longer recognize the person that is looking back at us, or that barely even fits in the mirror.

Whatever the reason, many of us wait until way too late—until after a major health crisis arises—to get serious about taking care of our bodies' health. From the moment you start your first fast, however, you begin rediscovering the discipline you may have learned as a child or teen, but have set aside, in some aspects of your life. And by the end of your first successful fast, even if it lasts only a day, you will have found how good it feels to take back some control over your life. Try it, you'll see!

Benefit from a Short and Easy Fast

Arguably, a one-day fast is also the most versatile kind. While many people ultimately go on to longer fasts, I have noticed that a significant number of fasters tend to stick with the 24-hour option. I attribute most of the reasons to its versatility and practicality:

- Saves time
- Requires little preparation
- Can result in weight loss (if done on alternate days)

First, you don't have to clear out a block of time for a one-day fast. Do it on a day when either you're not working or you have a light load, or perhaps on a weekend day when the weather forecast calls for cold wind or rain, which means that in all likelihood you'll be sticking close to home anyway. A 14-day fast, by contrast, takes much more advance planning. Depending on your personality and physical strength, to say nothing of your work or family situation, a long fast can and often does lead to a major rearranging of your normal activities.

Second, there is minimal preparation involved in a one-day fast, and ending a fast this short is comparatively simple and trouble free. Plus, when you fast for only a day, you can significantly increase the frequency. Some people will juice fast one day every week—that's 52 healing days a year!—while others, particularly those interested in losing some poundage, will fast on alternate days for a given period...say, over a span of 10 days to 2 weeks.

A third reason is that, since you can lose a pound a day on a juice fast, doing an alternate-day fast is an extremely good way to drop some of your unwanted weight. Keep in mind, though, that this will work *only* if you eat moderately on your nonfasting days, and even then rely heavily on fruits and vegetables, with some fish, eggs, or chicken for both variety and protein. Don't try to make up lost calories on those days when you do eat, because if that's your inclination, alternate-day fasting will be a waste of time from the standpoint of shedding weight.

DON'T FRET ABOUT YOUR PROTEIN

The importance of protein in the human diet cannot be denied—but it's also important to realize that protein is available in many fruits and vegetables. As an example, USDA Handbook No. 456, *Nutritive Value of American Foods in Common Units*, lists these protein percentages in plant foods:

- Spinach, 49 percent
- Broccoli, 45 percent
- Lettuce, 34 percent
- Cabbage, 22 percent
- Lemons, 16 percent
- Oranges, 8 percent
- Watermelon, 8 percent
- Grapes, 8 percent

Many other fruits and vegetables contain protein as well. But if you're juice fasting and think that you need still more protein, then simply add a daily teaspoon of high-quality protein power to one of your juice concoctions.

In any event, a one-day fast—whether it's done once a year, once a week, or every other day for a short period —does good things for your overall health and will give your immune system *and* your life a definite energy boost.

Do a Two-Day Fast...or a Longer One

The next level of juice fasting is a two-day fast, often referred to as a "weekend fast" (since this is the time frame most people will choose). Fasting over the weekend makes a lot of sense. If you start your fast on Friday evening, after you've had time to get home from work, unwind a bit (but not with an alcoholic beverage), and eat a leisurely dinner, then you can end it on Sunday evening, have another leisurely dinner, and get up for work Monday morning refreshed and energized and ready to charge into the week. And believe me, you will be feeling better than many of your friends and coworkers—at least, those who spent the weekend enjoying a cocktail or three and dining on their regular fare. Actually, you'll be feeling *much* better than them.

A two-day fast and a three-day fast generally accomplish the same things: They give your body a break from its regular routine, and they get your health pointed back in the right direction. Energy that your body normally would use for digestion and metabolism is instead made available for repair of inflamed cells and for miscellaneous clean-up duties. This is why a two-day fast and a three-day fast are commonly, and collectively, called *rejuvenation fasts*. Your body is silently doing the general housecleaning that you, as a homeowner, might do around the house over a two- or three-day weekend.

You may notice that I keep drawing comparisons between fasting and cleaning your home or office. Though that admittedly sounds a bit trite, it is also exceedingly accurate. I'm hoping that these comparisons will give you a better mental picture of what fasting can accomplish, as opposed to my using more-technical terms that many would find tedious or even baffling.

Shorter Fasts Can Be a Real Challenge

Many readers of this book might not believe what I'm about to say, but a two- or three-day fast can actually be the most difficult fasts of all, especially for first-timers. This is because the second and third days of *any* fast are usually the most difficult. Two or three days are the time frame in which your body adjusts, from running on the calories it normally receives through the meals and snacks you eat, to using the resources that it has already processed and stored away.

During the first two to three days of a fast, most people will also experience a feeling of emptiness—you might call it hunger—since you are no longer filling your stomach constantly. Then, I must point out, there is a psychological component too, which will be covered in some detail in Chapter 6. For now, though, let me say that the psychological or emotional pressures that fasting sometimes causes are felt most strongly by people who eat for comfort—that is, those of us who use food to relieve the stresses of our daily life rather than as tools to detox and rebuild our cells and to gain energy to achieve our goals.

Regardless, though, by Day 4 of a longer fast, virtually everyone has gotten past these initial, and generally slight, feelings of discomfort. At that point, juice fasting almost always becomes easy as pie, because once your body has had time to adjust to these new circumstances it will switch over to automatic pilot and get busy cleaning and restoring itself, like one of those trendy little vacuums that robotically clean the floor.

Longer Fasts Can Perform Some Deep Cleansing

By Day 7 of a fast, your body has transitioned into a deep cleansing mode, and now it's seriously gearing up to rid your body of years of accumulated toxins. Your liver has begun to seriously purge itself. All manner of nasty chemical and poisons—from food preservatives and pesticides to air pollutants that have entered through your lungs—are being drawn out of your cells and poured into your bloodstream, bile, sweat, or urine for elimination. Other fasting experts have said that, at this point, your body is "battling the pollutants as if you had just consumed them." I fully agree. (To give a nasty example, what do you do moments after you mistakenly eat some spoiled food? You throw it up! That's your body taking care of you, with no "thinking" involved.)

As you move past Day 7 and head toward completing a two-week fast, or one that's even longer, you will notice still more dramatic changes beginning to occur. You are now in the realm of *deep tissue cleansing,* in which the debris in your blood and lymphatic fluid is being filtered out and disposed of and your organs are beginning to regenerate. This is a pretty heady time in any fast, and the feelings that may come over you can range from euphoria and excitement to distress and irritability (more on this in Chapter 6). Most people report good feelings during this time, rather than bad.

Caution: Here I must mention one thing about lengthy fasts—you need to fall into one of the following categories (or into both of them) before you undertake a fast lasting seven days or more:

- You are an experienced faster who understands exactly what is involved and what you'll be getting into, *and/or*
- You are being guided by a medical or naturopathic professional with knowledge of fasting, as well as first-hand experience.

If you observe this caution, then I assure you that you can fast comfortably on fresh juice for as long as your body itself remains at ease with the fast.

Juice-Fasting Programs

While fasting on juices, you need to aim to drink 60 to 90 ounces (about 7 to 11 eight-ounce glasses) of raw juice over any 24-hour period, depending on your weight and age. For those with a sensitive stomach, it is best to dilute the pure juice 50 percent with purified water. On all these fasting programs, aim to drink 20 to 30 ounces (2½ to 3½ glasses) of water during any 24-hour period. If you get bloated, you can dilute the raw juice further or reduce the quantity of juice you are drinking.

Morning, mid-day, and evening, drink as much of the 30 ounces of juice as you feel like, then drink the rest over the next few hours. (Few people can chug down 30 ounces at one time.) Some people like to set a timer in their kitchen or on their computer, reminding them to drink 5 or 6 ounces every waking hour (*plus* the water, in between).

You might want to keep a little notebook log of each drink, to keep track of your daily volume.

If you become super-busy, remember that you can freeze the juice immediately after making it, take it with you as you go about your day, and then drink it after it thaws out.

For ease of use, the juice combinations that I refer to in the programs below are listed by number in Chapter 7 (see pages 110–127).

One-Day Energy Fast

The one-day energy fast is possibly the most popular fast of all, for the simple reason that it is easy and convenient and will fit into almost any schedule—yet offers a number of healthy benefits. A one-day fast, for example, helps you control your desire for unhealthy foods while allowing your body to rest some of its systems and focus instead on repair and cleaning. As for the "energizing" effects of a one-day fast, these will come primarily from your choice of juices. Here, I would recommend that you start the day with an 8-ounce glass of pure water that contains the juice of 1 lime or ½ a lemon, and then over the course of the day enjoy the following three juice combinations:

• Morning: #37 (about 30 ounces)

• Noon: #38 (about 30 ounces)

• Night: #47 (about 30 ounces)

If you want to kick-start your one-day fast with an extra boost of energy, do five minutes of light stretches as soon as you get out of bed, followed by 60 seconds of deep breathing, and then drink your glass of water with lime or lemon juice. Next, take a walk of 30 minutes or more before having the day's first glass of fresh, raw juice. Follow this plan and I can guarantee that it won't be long until you experience a higher energy level.

Note: It is important to remember that the juice combinations I recommend are my personal favorites—the juices that I know will provide an energy boost. If you have come up with other juice combinations that seem energizing to you, or if you have a medical condition that would benefit from a particular juice combination, then by all means make a substitution. This is about your health, and not anyone else's.

Two-Day Detox Fast

My personal favorite fast is a two-day detoxification fast. It is very convenient (it can be done over a two-day weekend, so it won't interfere with work or school), while also offering some fairly substantial health benefits. On this fast, for 48 hours *your body* has a break from "normal" activities such as digesting food and storing all manner of nasty toxins. In their place it can concentrate on replacing damaged cells and getting rid of the harmful herbicides and pesticides—as well as a wide range of other damaging chemicals—that most of us regularly ingest.

I'd be the first to tell you that a two-day detox fast isn't going to reverse years of toxin-related damage. Still, it's a good

and healthy first step in that reversal process. Restoring anything that has been damaged—a car, a house, a valuable paint-
ing, your body—isn't going to happen overnight. But you have
to start somewhere, and on each day of a two-day detox fast
I'd start with a 5-to-10-minute full-body massage with a dry
brush (see page 89), followed by a hot bath or shower to stimulate the skin, open your pores, and get rid of toxins.

Then, I would look to my juicer to prepare the following
detox drinks:

DAY ONE
• Morning: #5 (about 30 ounces)
• Noon: #18 (about 30 ounces)
• Night: #30 (about 30 ounces)

DAY TWO
   Repeat Day One, *or:*
• Morning: #39 (about 30 ounces)
• Noon: #6 (about 30 ounces)
• Night: #42 (about 30 ounces)

Note: It is important to remember that the juice combinations I recommend are my personal favorites—the juices that
I've found to be very good at detoxing the body. If you have
come up with other juice combinations that are equally good,
or if you have a medical condition that would benefit from a
particular juice combination, then by all means make a substitution. This is about your health, and not anyone else's.

Three-Day Rejuvenation Fast

To rejuvenate, by definition, is to "make young or youthful
again," "to give new vigor to," and "to restore to the original
state." I am not so bold, or so foolish, as to claim that a three-
day rejuvenation fast with fresh fruit and vegetable juices will
totally rejuvenate your body, though in some cases it comes

close. But I will say with no hesitation that juice fasting *can* and *does* give you a new lease on life.

Like the two-day detox fast, a three-day rejuvenation fast allows your body to take a break from its everyday activities related to digesting food. In the place of these activities, your fasting body will focus on the same sort of general housekeeping and cleaning chores that you might undertake in your own home if it had been neglected for a while or was particularly dirty after a prolonged visit by your children or grandchildren.

A three-day rejuvenation fast, whether it's done as a stand-alone fast or as one of a series of three-day fasts, will in and of itself give new vigor to your body. I recommend, however, that you supplement your fast with a daily sauna or steam bath and regular exercise, which can be anything from a walk around the neighborhood to time spent pulling weeds in the garden or cleaning out the garage.

For this particular fast, I recommend six different juice combinations (60 to 90 ounces each day):

#8, #29, #33, #34, #37, #42

I believe that with a fast of any length, you should drink fresh, raw juice a minimum of three times a day: morning, noon, and night. And you should also drink various combinations of juices to ensure that (a) you don't become bored with juicing and (b) you get all the essential vitamins and minerals that your body requires. But, obviously, I can't expect most juice fasters to find and purchase enough different fruits and vegetables to drink a different combo three (or more) times a day for a long period. So, if your juice fast is going to extend beyond a couple of days, but will last less than a week, I'd suggest finding four to six recipes that will meet your body's needs, as well as appeal to your taste buds, and then alternate the recipes throughout the duration of the fast. A juice fast can be the healthiest thing going, but if it's not practical most people will give it up—and sooner rather than later.

Note: It is important to remember that the juice combinations I recommend are my personal favorites—the juices that I've found to be very good at rejuvenating the body. If you have come up with other juice combinations that are equally good, or if you have a medical condition that would benefit from a particular juice combination, then by all means make a substitution. This is about your health, and not anyone else's.

Seven-Day Deep Cleanse Fast

In most respects, seven consecutive days of drinking nothing but raw fruit and vegetable juices (don't forget your water!) provides the full spectrum of juice-fasting benefits. Your body has ample time to detoxify. A full 168 consecutive hours are devoted to replacing and repairing damaged tissue. The length of the fast offers ample time for complementary therapies, which (depending on your personal preferences) can include a colon cleansing, Epsom salt baths, body wraps, saunas and steam baths, mineral baths, or cider vinegar baths (see pages 87–90). The choice is yours—though I do suggest that everyone embarking on a seven-day fast have his or her colon cleansed on Day 2. There are several ways to go about this, from having a colonic done by a professional, to taking a home enema for three consecutive days, to using a herbal laxative. Again, the choice is yours.

Also, a seven-day fast is long enough to give your body a thorough respite from everyday digestive activities as well as provide plenty of time for the repair and replacement of damaged tissue. And at the same time, a seven-day fast is a realistic goal for almost anyone who desires a healthier body and already has a couple of shorter fasts under his or her belt.

As I said when discussing the three-day rejuvenation fast, I believe that with a fast of any length you should drink fresh, raw juice a minimum of three times a day: morning, noon, and night. And you should also drink various combinations of juices to ensure that (a) you don't become bored with juicing and (b) you get all the essential vitamins and minerals your body requires.

But, obviously, I can't expect most people to find and purchase enough different fruits and vegetables to drink a different combo three (or more) times a day for a long period. So, if your juice fast is going to extend to seven days or longer, I'd suggest finding an adequate number of recipes that meet your body's needs, as well as appeal to your taste buds, and alternate those recipes throughout the duration of the fast. A juice fast can be the healthiest thing going, but if it's not practical most people will give it up—and sooner rather than later.

For the seven-day deep cleanse fast, I recommend the following juice combinations (60 to 90 ounces each day):

#15, #17, #19, #30, #34, #39, #42, #43, #47, #48, #59

Note: It is important to remember that the juice combinations I recommend are my personal favorites—the juices that I find to be very good at giving the body a deep cleansing. If you have come up with other juice combinations that are equally good, or if you have a medical condition that would benefit from a particular juice combination, then by all means make a substitution. This is about your health, and not anyone else's.

Try Other Beneficial Practices, as Well

By now, you know that a primary benefit of fasting is ridding the body of toxic and dangerous wastes. As I mentioned early on, the colon and the skin are two of the main elimination pathways for such elimination. As a point of interest, approximately one-third of your body's impurities and waste are eliminated through the skin, with most of the rest leaving via the colon. For this reason, it is vital that you keep both systems working—and doing so effectively—during a fast of longer than two days. For a one- or two-day fast, you should experience no problems, but you may want to still consider what I'm about to say.

Cleaning Your Colon

A necessary part of your fast is cleansing your colon. When you stop eating solid food, the food that's already in your colon has nothing coming behind it to push it out. That is an oversimplification of the actual process, of course, but it simply means that the food remaining in the colon can go on to putrefy, which, in turn, creates toxins in your body. That's precisely *not* the thing you want at a time when you're trying to detoxify yourself!

To correct the situation, and to empty your colon and bowels, you have several different options, all of them good. Just select the one that you will be most comfortable with or is the most practical, taking into account your personal circumstances and feelings about these things.

Option 1: Make an appointment with a colon therapist, preferably for Day 2 of your fast, and have them do a colonic, or a thorough cleansing of the colon. This is the quickest solu-

tion, and for many people the easiest. To find a colon therapist, look in your local phone book or an alternative health
magazine. Many health-food stores also post this type of information on their bulletin boards or websites.

Option 2: If, for some reason—say, you live in a remote
area, it costs too much for your budget, it might embarrass
you—a colonic is not for you, then you can give yourself a
daily enema for three consecutive days, also beginning on Day
2 of the fast. At your local drugstore or discount store, you
can buy everything you need to self-administer an enema in
the privacy of your home; the package will even come with
instructions for use. Once you overcome any mental barriers
you may have erected as regards an enema, you'll find the
experience to be painless as well as very effective.

Option 3: Use an herbal laxative. Any quality health-food
store will have several brands in stock, and maybe even have
some advice to give you. Though this is not the option I
would recommend for most people, if it is the one you feel will
work best for you, then by all means let it be the one you use.

The bottom line here, and no pun intended, is that if you are
going to fast for longer than a day or two, you need to cleanse
your colon. Failing to do so probably won't cause you any
immediate harm, but the likelihood of health problems in the

DO ENEMAS SPARINGLY

A word of warning: It's a bad idea to fall into the habit of taking
an enema more than is absolutely necessary—whether for reasons of health, such as to alleviate acute constipation, or to
clean your colon during a fast. To do so puts you at risk of
weakening the natural defecation process and potentially creat-
ing a serious long-term problem. But for purposes of fasting
only, enemas are perfectly safe.

---

long run will increase proportionately to the length of your fast and the quantity of toxins that remain in your body—toxins that a good colon cleansing would expel.

Cleaning Your Skin

Keeping your skin clean and your pores wide open during a fast is another way to speed the elimination process and make it work as efficiently as possible. Actually, whenever you're fasting, skin cleansing is even more important than normal, because the chemicals and other toxins that will be discharged through your skin can cause everything from boils and pimples to rashes. Body odor can also be a bigger problem than usual.

The good news here is that there are quite a few easy, healthy, and enjoyable ways to keep your skin clean and breathing fully. You can start by just adding a dry-brush massage to your daily shower or bath routine. Acquire a natural bristle brush (not plastic!) with a long handle, and give yourself a 5-to-10-minute, full-body massage just before bathing or showering; do not scrub the skin roughly, just stimulate its blood flow. This is one of the simplest detox treatments, yet it is a highly effective way of stimulating your skin *and* encouraging the expulsion of toxins.

As a tip for women, some reports say that dry brushing will also help break down cellulite.

Other options for cleansing the skin and opening your pores include the following:

- Epsom salt baths, which promote perspiration and are excellent for helping you sweat our toxins
- A massage followed by an Epsom salt bath (2 cups to a tub of bath water), to deeply cleanse the skin by sloughing off old and dead cells (not for people with heart trouble or diabetes)

- Body wraps, which work like a sauna and help you eliminate toxic waste through sweating
- Saunas and steam baths; again, perspiration will carry toxins out of your body and skin
- Mineral baths, using mineral preparations available from any quality health-food store (directions will be on the label)
- Cider vinegar baths (2 cups of cider vinegar to a tub of warm water), which serve a dual purpose because they can also soothe itchy skin

My final recommendation here is to get outdoors whenever possible. Soak up some sunlight. Breathe in some fresh air (provided that the air is indeed fresh where you live). This is a healthy combination that will help your skin, as well as calm your soul, and will take the joy of living up a notch—whether or not you are fasting.

6

Handling Your Fast Well

Imagine for a moment that you were once a shiny new car, fresh off the showroom floor and firing on all cylinders, as close to perfection as you'd ever be and ready to hit the open road and discover what's around the next curve. Fine-tune this image just a bit and that new car could be a slightly younger version of yourself, ready to accelerate up and down the highway of life and into an exciting future full of good health.

Unfortunately, that may have been several hundred thousand miles ago...several hundred thousand *hard* miles ago, with a few wrong turns or smash-ups along the way. Today, aside from a few dents and a couple of dings, your body (car or otherwise) may still resemble that brand-new model, but the passing years and a general lack of maintenance have likely taken a heavy toll on most of the internal parts. Pistons and gears no longer work so well. Dirty oil. Squeaky door hinges. Road grime over everything. Clogged fuel injectors. Toxic waste and pollution—all have done a number on you.

The only solution, if you want a return to your pristine showroom form, is to carefully clean all your parts, from the biggest to the smallest, and hope that it's not too late—that no permanent damage was done. Likewise, the human body—your body!—also needs a periodic cleaning. The grime and pollution of daily living affects more than just cars. The best possible way to accomplish this cleaning on yourself is by juice fasting with fresh and raw juices from fruits and vegetables. As with your car, you'll want to start the restoration process before permanent damage sets in.

In fact, if you'll allow me to stick with this image for a moment longer, juice fasting not only can help you get back the speed and power of your younger years, but if you fast often enough, and follow my advice on your journey, it might even help you reach the point where that old family sedan (namely, you) starts to resemble a much newer, and perhaps even sportier, model. To arrive at this point, however, you must prepare for an occasional speed bump down the road—and having said that, I now promise you: no more metaphors.

I also need to remind you that each and every one of us is different, and that every single person who completes a juice fast will have his or her own personal and individual reactions to the experience. To be sure, lots of similarities will be noted, but even the similarities will be somewhat distinct. This means that everything you read in this book about the effects of fasting—and well as everything your friends might tell you or that you might read somewhere else—must be taken with a grain of salt, or, in this particular case, with a glass of juice (that's a fasting joke).

Understand the Effects of a Fast

The reason I'm asking you to keep this in mind is this: A fast will affect you, to a greater or lesser extent, in two quite different ways: physiological, which is how your body will react and change, and psychological, or how your mind will view the fast itself and also react to your physical changes and its *own* changes. In turn, your overall response to these body/mind changes may go a long way toward determining several things:

- The length of your fast
- The success of your fast
- Whether you ever fast again

Anyone who is familiar with my books knows that I try to avoid long and technical—and, therefore, usually boring—scientific explanations of how the body and its various organs and systems react to different circumstances, from diseases to cleansing programs. This information is readily available to anyone, so if that's your interest I recommend that you fire up a good Internet search engine or stop in at your local library. My personal feeling about this is that if I wanted to put you to sleep, I'd simply recommend that you ask your doctor for a sleeping pill.

In the case of juice fasting, the physical and psychological effects will be determined, in large part, by precisely how toxic your body is. If you are relatively young, were raised a vegetarian, have avoided most or all processed foods, and live far from the smog and pollution of a large city or manufacturing center, then you may already be free of most toxins—and, lucky you, you may experience only a few symptoms of detoxification during your fast.

If, by contrast, you have lived your entire life near a freeway or an industrial complex, take most or all of your meals at fast-food restaurants, and enjoy spending your spare time sipping cocktails in smoke-filled bars, then you are probably a walking toxic-waste dump. On a juice fast, you may come face-to-face with some potentially severe symptoms as your body detoxifies itself and attempts to regain a healthy footing.

Either way, however, juice fasting will provide some definite, health-related benefits—what they consist of will be a matter of degree. And, frankly, most of us badly need to undergo detoxification. Exactly what you can expect from it is, again, an individual thing.

Fasting's Physiological Effects

Speaking in general terms, the average person undertaking a juice fast of three to seven days, or longer, might experience one or more of the following reactions:

- Dizziness
- Headache
- Lightheadedness
- Skin rashes
- Lower-than-normal blood pressure
- Normalization of high blood pressure
- Elimination of mucus from the chest, throat, and nose
- Increased urinary output
- Strong odor to the urine
- Smelly bowel movements
- Elimination of parasites from the bowel
- Elimination of gallstones from the biliary tract (these are sometimes even seen in bowel movements)
- Tiredness
- Constipation
- Diarrhea
- Abdominal cramps
- Nausea
- Increased body odor

- Bad breath
- Coated tongue
- Weight loss
- Loss of cellulite

These are just the physical symptoms (we'll touch on psychological in a moment). For most everyone, they will usually be mild and pass very quickly.

However—and this is terribly important—if you experience the side effects I have listed, or any others, and they get worse over time instead of better, then by all means stop your fast immediately and, if necessary, seek the appropriate medical attention. As I stated in Chapter 4, fasting is extremely safe 99.99 percent of the time *if* you are a fairly healthy person

---

HOW TO RELIEVE SYMPTOMS

On a juice fast, your body might go several days to a week or more before you have a physical reaction to the detox process—or you could see a detox reaction on the first day of your fast. This varies greatly from person to person, as do the types of possible reactions. The most likely detox reactions are occasional nausea, headache, and weakness or tiredness.

For nausea, I've found that nutmeg or lemon balm (*Melissa officinalis*, in the mint family), mixed into a glass of juice, will usually relieve the problem. Many juice fasters have gotten relief from nausea by juicing parsley leaves with their other fruits and vegetables.

Celery juice and fennel juice are both good remedies if you're experiencing a detox-related headache. As for relieving the weakness and tiredness that may accompany a detoxifying juice fast, do the same things you'd do if you weren't fasting: take a nap if you're at home, or take a few deep breaths, stretch, and wash your face if you're not.

Daily life when you're juice fasting is, in one respect, not that much different from your nonfasting life. Common sense will usually save the day.

---

with a good perspective on what a fast entails. But we cannot and must not forget about that other 0.01 percent. If you find that you fall into this category, and I certainly hope that you don't, then it's imperative that you not let fasting make you ill or otherwise compromise your health.

So, please, whenever you fast, always listen attentively to what your body is telling you and then act, and react, accordingly.

If all this talk of "symptoms" and "side effects" and such is getting you down, then stop right now and consider the following: For 99.99 percent of the population, these are actually good and positive things. Sure, a very few people might experience some temporary discomfort from time to time during a fast, but all this means is that their body has gone on the toxin warpath and is doing its best to cleanse itself and expel the nasty pollutants that contribute to an entire spectrum of health problems, from cancer to arthritis. If you've ever played sports, you've likely heard a coach say something to the effect of "No pain, no gain"…well, that can apply to fasting, too, though the majority of people can replace "pain" with "slight discomfort." And believe me, the discomfort of fasting will be significantly less than the great gain.

But—one more time—if a fast ever becomes too uncomfortable, or too painful in any way, discontinue it immediately. You need not feel any shame in doing so; in truth, the mere fact that you began a fast in the first place means that you have more mental strength and more determination than most people around you. Always be proud of what you've accomplished, and never chastise yourself or feel let down or embarrassed if health concerns require you to cut a fast short. This is the doctor in me speaking, as well as the friend to all fasters.

Fasting's Psychological Effects

On the psychological side of the fasting coin, many people will experience an occasional valley (low point), but it has been my experience that peaks (high points) are much more common. And for quite a few people the mental low points don't occur at all—with two noticeable exceptions. Those are what I like to call the *My Stomach Feels Empty* syndrome and the *My Mouth Wants to Chew* syndrome.

Man or woman, humans were made to eat. Eating is generally a good thing, as long as we choose the right foods—something that many of us have a big problem with. When we fail to choose the right foods enough of the time, our bodies become overloaded with toxins. We can easily reach a point at which our good health requires a juice fast.

(Obviously, now, the preceding paragraph doesn't apply to everyone. There are those among us who consciously avoid most toxins and therefore fast with juices only because they want to make their healthy bodies even healthier. These folks may be in a minority, but they do exist.)

The average person, under normal circumstances, will eat two or three full meals a day, supplemented by one or more between-meal snacks. This is a habit the majority of us picked up in childhood, and one that's been part of our lives ever since. Many of us will even have a late-night snack that follows on the heels of a full dinner—and if you are one of those people, and if you are also in the habit of eating breakfast, then your stomach will likely feel full, or partially so, from the time you rise in the morning to the time you go to bed at night.

Your stomach, in essence, is never going to feel truly empty, except perhaps during the middle of the night—when you're asleep and therefore totally unaware of the feeling. But this will all change when you start a fast. Somewhere between three to five hours after your last meal or that final snack, your stomach will start to feel a little hollow and "wonder" what happened to its supply of food. A signal will go out to your brain, saying: "It's time to eat! Hurry, where's my food?" Only you can't eat—because you're fasting...remember?

Over the course of the next day or so, these stomach-to-brain signals—which are often referred to as plain old hunger pangs—may well intensify. And your brain, tired of the constant nagging, will probably start telling you that your stomach needs filling. The *My Stomach Feels Empty* syndrome has once again reared its hungry head. Ignore its message! It will soon go away. As I've discussed, most people won't feel hunger after the third day of a fast, and many will get over the feeling even sooner. Besides, it's an easy thing to ignore...believe me, it is.

From time to time, I've asked some of my patients a question like this: "How many people do you personally know, or have heard of, who've died or been hospitalized or otherwise been hindered in their daily activities by feeling a little bit hungry—not starving, but just feeling hungry?" The answer, as you might imagine, is always, "Well, none." Case closed, Judge Cabot!

Potentially more distressing to many people is the *My Mouth Wants to Chew* syndrome, which also covers the sensation of taste. Tasting will not be a problem on a juice fast—as opposed to a water fast—since few things are more delicious than fresh fruit and vegetable juices. A lot of people, though, do seem to miss chewing; to them, it's almost a habit, like breathing is an involuntary instinct, and they miss it when it stops.

Lest you think I'm crazy for saying this, consider that roughly a third of all adults in the United States are overweight—and the problem is getting worse. A team of researchers at Johns Hopkins University in Baltimore pre-dicted that if people kept gaining weight at the 2007 rate, excess body fat would be the *norm* by 2015, with an astonishing 75 percent of U.S. adults overweight and 41 percent qualifying as obese. And according to U.S. govern-ment statistics, 16 percent of U.S. children are already overweight—and more than twice that many percent are at risk of becoming overweight.

Obesity is a complex public health crisis, but the reason so many people are overweight is quite simple: They eat too often, and when they do eat, they eat too much. Now, suppose for a moment that food was absorbed through the skin...that you could just hold a piece of pie in your hand and all the fat and calories would somehow be absorbed. It sounds ludi-crous, I know, but if that were the way your body worked, do you think so many of us would be fat? I seriously doubt it!

I find it unlikely that you would miss the feeling of absorption (if you could even feel it in the first place). Chewing, though, is another matter altogether.

I'm convinced that putting food in your mouth, tasting it, chewing it up, and swallowing it can become every bit as addictive and as comforting as nicotine or alcohol. So, for some people, starting a fast can be as difficult—both physi-cally and mentally—as giving up cigarettes or not having a drink. The *My Mouth Wants to Chew* syndrome is quite real, and something you need to be aware of before you begin a fast. Luckily, it is also easy to overcome. All it takes is a touch of determination, plus a pinch of willpower.

Aside from these two syndromes (which, of course, I made up for purposes of illustration), the mental side of fasting is relatively benign for most of us. Mental highs, as I've said, are the most obvious and the most consistent psychological effect.

These highs are quite pleasant and a nice side benefit, so to speak, of the fasting process itself.

I once read an Internet posting from an unidentified source, who quoted another writer/author (also unnamed) as saying:

> You will notice that during fasting your mental perception and awareness will be sharpened and that your thoughts will gradually rise from an everyday level of unpleasant realities to higher realities, concerned with the purpose and meaning of your life. Your heart will rejoice, your problems will seem unimportant, and you'll feel happy to be alive. And you will be amazed how your mental activity will be sharpened and how thoughts and new ideas will flow with ease. All in all, your fasting will be a wonderful experience, which will recharge, renew and rejuvenate your whole personality—body, mind and spirit.

I wish I knew the identity of the person who wrote this. Whoever he or she is has my gratitude, for the writer obviously knows first-hand the power of fasting and how it can transform the entire person, not merely the body itself. This is indeed a message worth sharing, and I hope to carry on that sharing in the final chapters of this book.

Find Answers to Frequently Asked Questions

Whenever I discuss the effects of fasting with patients or friends, they typically pepper me with a number of questions. In thinking back on our dialogues, I've discovered that many of these questions are fairly similar, or sometimes even identical. I suspect, therefore, that a lot of you reading this book may have some of the same questions, too. Let me answer a few.

Should I Be Concerned About Fasting's Side Effects?

Q. I've heard about many of the unpleasant side effects of fasting, such as bad breath and skin problems, but I don't quite understand the cause. Could you explain this a little better?

A. The majority of the toxins—chemical additives, preservatives, plastics, solvents, pesticides, herbicides, and so on—that have accumulated in your body over your lifetime are stored in body fat. When you stop eating, your body turns to these fat cells and starts burning them for energy, and as this occurs the stored toxins are released into your bloodstream. This process ultimately results in the toxins' being expelled through organs such as the liver, the kidneys, the intestines, the lungs, and the skin. So, it's pretty understandable—don't you think?—that poisons exiting the body through your skin could cause a rash, while pollutants expelled via the lungs might leave your breath a little less than sweet. An explicit scientific explanation would be more complicated, of course, but the short answer here is this: *All* physical reactions to fasting are the direct result of accumulated toxins being pulled out of storage, and then being kicked out of your body through one or more organs. And as I've previously said, these symptoms and side effects, though they might be unpleasant at the time, are always temporary and should be seen as a positive sign, since they signify that your body is cleansing and repairing itself.

Can a First-Timer Like Me Succeed?

Q. Are most people able to successfully complete a fruit and vegetable juice fast the very first time they try?

A. More than anything else, my answer to this question depends on the length of your initial fast. If you are talking about a one-day fast, then I would certainly say "yes." I would give the same answer about a two-day fast. But if you're talking about a first fast of a week or longer, then I'd have to say that a significant number of people—possibly even the majority—would break their fast before it's over, simply because of the newness of the experience and the physical difficulties (real or perceived) that are involved. You have to understand that there are no hard and fast statistics on this; there is no official "fasting record keepers," the way there are in all sports leagues. Based on my own observations, though, I'd say that if successfully completing your first fast is all-important to you, then start with a fast of only one or two days. The reason: The longer you go, the more difficult it's going to be, especially the first time around. It is my opinion, too, that the truly important thing you need to understand here is that fasting is not about ego or about bragging rights, or anything like that. *It's about improving your health.* If you forget this—if you place more value on "winning" than on "trying"—then your fasting priorities are definitely misplaced.

How Would I Handle Tiredness?

Q. I've heard that sometimes when you fast, you get really tired. Is this true, and if it is what can I do about it?

A. For some people, this will be true—you will feel a lot more tired than you normally do. This feeling may pass in a short time (say, a few minutes to an hour), or it might last for a day or more. Again, it depends on the individual, since fasting can and will affect everyone differently. If you happen to experience a level of tiredness that starts to feel unacceptable, or if it truly begins to interfere with your daily activities, you can try one of several countermeasures. First, make sure that you are getting an adequate amount of fresh fruit and vegetable juices. We'll discuss recommended daily quantities in Chapter 7, so here I'll just say that as you get into a fast and your appetite begins to wane, you may find yourself, consciously or unconsciously, cutting back on the volume of juice you are drinking. Don't let this happen! Stick with my recommendations and make sure you drink an appropriate amount of juice at regular intervals throughout the day. Also, don't just find one or two juices you like and stick with those, day after day. It's important to mix it up. Combine the juices of fruits with the juices of vegetables and fresh herbs. Continue to experiment. One of the great advantages of raw juice fasting over other types of fasting is that juice fasting can give you all the vitamins and minerals you need to stay healthy, so long as you juice adequate amounts of several types of both fruits and vegetables every day. If for some reason you still feel that you are not getting enough vitamins and minerals, you can also take a multivitamin/mineral supplement, though I don't actually recommend this. I've found that for some people, taking a pill on an empty stomach can cause a little upset, and a number of vitamins and supplements cannot be properly used by the body unless taken with foods. Finally, you can always try something that usually works when you are tired but not fasting: Take a nap, for example, or have a massage.

What if I Feel I Have to Eat Something?

Q. What should I do if I'm in the middle of a fast and really want to see it through to the end, but feel that I absolutely have to have something to eat? Should I just quit the fast, or is it OK to eat a small meal?

A. That's a great question. The situation you describe is one that many first-time fasters will face. I have two answers. First, I'd recommend that you try everything and anything you can think of to get over this particular hump without eating. You can always try increasing the amount of water you are drinking, as this often helps alleviate the empty, "hollow" feeling that passes for hunger. Or maybe you could get around this feeling by reading an exciting or a comforting book, talking to a friend, playing with the cat, or taking a walk or a jog. Imagine what you would do to pick yourself up or distract yourself if you were feeling a little blue or wanted to stop worrying about something, and then try that. Getting through an especially bad bout of hunger will always be easier said than done, but I promise you it *can* be done; I know this first-hand. A second approach, if your feelings of hunger become so overwhelming that you know you're positively going to quit the fast unless you have a snack, is to eat a piece or two of apple and a small quantity of salad vegetables, all raw. A cup of freshly made tomato or vegetable soup makes a good choice, too. These are the sorts of foods you would be eating to break a completed fast, so these are also the best options for a mid-fast snack. In any event, do not overeat, and be sure to chew the apple and vegetables extremely well. I've never seen any problems result from having this type of snack during a juice fast. Still, don't interrupt your fast like this more than once. After all, one of fasting's main benefits is giving your digestive tract a good rest and allowing your body to concentrate on disposing of its load of toxins. If you continue to disrupt that process by eating, then you may as well end the fast, feel good about what you were able to accomplish, and concentrate on doing a little better the next time.

Can I Stay on a Fast, Even Though I Smoke?

Q. I don't like to admit it, but I'm a smoker. Will this make fasting more difficult?

A. Sure it will. In fact, it will initially make it much more difficult. Not only will you be giving up food, which for many of us is an addiction itself, but you'll also be trying to control a second addiction at the same time—assuming that you remain strong during the fast and stay away from your cigarettes (or cigars or pipe). Common sense should tell you that "2 X difficult = *more* difficult." Still, you shouldn't let a little obstacle stand in your way, because the reward of completing a fast, while simultaneously kicking an extremely bad habit, will be twice as great. It has been my experience, and others say the same, that fasting can actually help you move away from destructive cravings. It does so first by eliminating the accumulated toxins within your body that can cause those cravings. Then, if you continue with fasting, it helps your reserves of willpower and determination to grow, thus enabling you to better fight your desire for unhealthy and unnatural substances, among which tobacco is one of the worst. It's important to keep in mind, too, that a juice fast will make you feel so much healthier, and so much better about yourself, that those good feelings will naturally encourage you to stay away from bad habits. So, if you are a smoker and want to fast and not smoke while fasting, go for it! It may take more than one fast to rid you of the habit, but if you keep trying, it won't be long until you are known as a former smoker.

As I near the end of this chapter on the physical, the psychological, and the overall effects of fasting, I'd be remiss if I didn't mention one final benefit: the spiritual effect. Regardless of which God, or god, you may believe in, or even if you believe in no deity or Higher Power at all, it's a fact that millions upon millions of people fast not only for better health but for spiritual illumination, as well. Fasting is mentioned in the

Christian Bible. Muslims, Hindus, and Jews all fast as part of their respective religions. Granted, in most cases we're not talking about juice fasting per se, but no matter. In this sense, fasting is fasting—and its spiritual rewards, which are an entirely individual thing, can be quite as powerful whether you totally abstain from water and juice, sustain yourself with just water, or choose to drink water and juice both.

Perhaps the best-known faster of all, at least to the world at large, was Mahatma Gandhi, who led a long, nonviolent movement for freedom in India, which was then under British control. It was he who reportedly told his followers, "The light of the world will illuminate within you when you fast and purify yourself." And, with that having been said, there is really nothing more to say.

7

Glorious Juice Recipes

The wise and compassionate father of modern-day medicine, Hippocrates, is supposed to have said something like the following:

> Everyone has a doctor in him or her; we just have to help it in its work. The natural healing force within each one of us is the greatest force in getting well. Our food should be our medicine. Our medicine should be our food.

Since Hippocrates died nearly 2,400 years ago, in 377 B.C., long before the invention of the electric juicing machine and at a time when many of today's fruits and vegetables were likely not available in his native Greece, it is doubtful that he was ever a "juice faster" in the present sense of that term. But I'll bet that he would be if he were alive in the 21st century—and reasonably so, given his philosophy of diet and medicine.

If it were up to me, juicing and regular fasting with raw fruit, vegetable, and fresh herb juices would be as common in modern medicine and in today's society as filling a prescription from your doctor or taking the family to eat at a fast-food restaurant. Everyone would do juicing—and everyone would be much healthier as a result. It's hard to say why more people, especially in developed countries, don't realize this. Maybe it's simply a matter of getting the word out.

I do know, however, that in the same way that the longest journey always begins with a single step, your personal journey toward a longer and healthier life can begin with your first juice fast. So, let me now officially welcome you to juice fasting and introduce you to some of my favorite—and most healing—juicing recipes.

As an added benefit, I am also listing some of the medical conditions and diseases that these recipes can help bring under control. So, when deciding which fruits and vegetables you would like to juice next, you can make your selection based not only on flavor, but on other health-related benefits as well.

Most of the recipes I've listed will give you 1 to 2 cups of juice, though there will always be variation. Some oranges, for instance, are juicier than others, depending on where they're grown, their type, the season, and so on. Everything from radishes and carrots to pears and apples can vary in size, which can and does affect juice content. The important thing here is to drink enough fresh juice every day to ensure that your body receives an adequate amount of vitamins and nutri-

---

WATER: YOU CAN'T GET ENOUGH OF IT

The problem of dehydration can easily be overcome by drinking six to eight 8-ounce glasses of water a day. I highly recommend this to every juice faster, regardless of their juice intake. Juice is delicious in most of its many combinations, but nothing works as well as water for quenching your thirst and keeping your body and its many organs—particularly the kidneys—well hydrated and functioning properly.

---

ents, as well as a sufficient amount of liquid. You definitely do *not* want to become dehydrated during your fast.

And if you discover that any of my juice recipes—or, indeed, juice recipes that you may find elsewhere in your reading in magazines or on the Internet—are a bit strong or overbearing for your taste, then just add a portion of that day's water supply. As a starting point, I suggest a mixture of 3 parts juice to 1 part water, but you can always deviate from this, to suit your personal preference and your fondness for specific flavors.

You are actually safe in drinking virtually any amount of juice on a daily basis. It has been my experience that your body will let you know when you have had enough. And, certainly, the bigger you are and the more you weigh, the more juice you'll likely drink. At any rate, I don't have a maximum daily recommendation, but I do recommend that you drink a minimum of 32 to 64 ounces (that's 4 to 8 glasses) of fresh juice each day during your fast. Again, a smaller person might be satisfied with 32 ounces—plus the recommended 48 to 64 ounces of water—while a larger person might well drink 64 or more ounces of juice in addition to the water. It's all about individual need and individual choice.

You'll find that the majority of my juice recipes below combine citrus with other fruits and vegetables. The reason for that? Overall, I have chosen ingredients for their taste as well as their therapeutic benefit. Even so, many people new to juice fasting may find that some of the flavors will initially pose a taste-bud challenge, so to speak. This is where the sunny, refreshing taste of citrus, especially oranges, can help. Oranges combine well with almost any vegetable, with carrots being a favorite companion juice.

A good beginner juice, and one that I've found that most people really enjoy, contains 2 oranges (peeled) and 2 carrots.

If this works well for you, then try adding a 1-inch slice of fresh pineapple. And from here, juicing is an open road, full of so many exciting and exotic flavors that no palate, no matter how particular, will be disappointed. So, let the juicing begin…with my reminder that I start every recipe with a medical condition (or two) that the particular juice combination may help prevent, control, or relieve.

Try These Delicious, Healthy Juices for Fasting and Daily Enjoyment

The recipe numbers below are given for ease of use only; there is no special significance to recipe order. (See page 85 for the various juice-fasting programs.)

1 GOOD FOR ANEMIA

2 oranges, peeled

2 spinach leaves

½ beetroot and tops

2 apricots, pitted

¼-ounce of fresh wheatgrass juice (optional)

Note: Wheatgrass requires a slow juice extractor; alternatively, it can be purchased at most health-food stores

2 GOOD FOR ARTHRITIS AND GOUT

1 grapefruit, peeled

1 cup cherries, pitted

4 stalks celery, leaves removed

1 sprig parsley

1-inch slice ginger root

2 carrots

3 GOOD FOR RHEUMATOID ARTHRITIS

1 lemon, peeled

1-inch slice fresh pineapple

1 clove garlic *or* 1-inch slice red onion

2 stalks celery, leaves removed

1 apple

½-inch slice ginger root

4 GOOD FOR ASTHMA AND LUNG WEAKNESS

1 orange, peeled

1 lemon, peeled

2 apricots, pitted

2 carrots

2 stalks celery, leaves removed

2 leaves spinach

¼-inch ginger root

1 handful mixed fresh herbs, chopped—lemon thyme,
    basil, cilantro, mint

5 GOOD FOR CANCER PREVENTION AND TREATMENT

2 oranges, with some peel

1 lemon, with some peel

1 carrot

½ red beetroot

1 clove garlic *or* 1-inch slice red onion

3 broccoli florets

1 handful mixed fresh herbs, chopped—parsley, basil,
    oregano, mint

Dilute with ½ cup strong green tea

6 GOOD FOR CANCER PREVENTION AND TREATMENT

2 oranges, peeled

½ papaya

½ beetroot and tops
½-inch slice ginger root
1 red radish
2 carrots
1 cup cabbage, chopped

7 GOOD FOR COLDS AND THE FLU
1 lemon, peeled
1 grapefruit, peeled
1 clove garlic *or* 1-inch slice red onion
½-inch slice ginger root
2 red apples, with skin
1 handful mixed fresh herbs, chopped—cilantro, thyme,
    oregano, parsley
Add 1 cup hot water and 1 Tbsp. honey

Sprinkle with cayenne pepper (*optional*)

8 HAS A SOOTHING EFFECT ON THE STOMACH AND
INTESTINES
2 oranges, peeled
2 red apples, peeled
2-inch slice fresh pineapple
3 stalks celery, leaves removed
¼ beetroot

9 HELPS FIGHT DEPRESSION
2 oranges, with some peel
1 carrot
¼ beetroot and tops
2-inch slice watermelon
½ cup fresh mint, chopped
Sprinkle with cayenne *or* hot sauce (*optional*)

10 HELPS WITH ANXIETY

2 oranges, peeled

1 carrot

6 strawberries

2 stalks celery, leaves removed

3 lettuce leaves

11 CAN HELP PREVENT DIABETES AND LOWER BLOOD
SUGAR

½ grapefruit, peeled but with pith left on

¼ bitter melon (if available) *or* 6 green string beans,
    chopped

½ carrot

2 stalks celery, leaves left on

2 dandelion leaves *or* 2 cabbage leaves

1 spring onion *or* ½ clove garlic

¼ cup fennel, chopped

Mix with ½ tsp. fenugreek powder steeped in ¼ cup
    hot water

12 REDUCES THE PAIN OF FIBROMYALGIA

1 orange, peeled

1 lemon, peeled

1 carrot

3 stalks celery, leaves removed

2 leaves spinach

1 cucumber, peeled

1-inch slice fresh ginger root

2-inch slice fresh pineapple

13 HELPS PREVENT OR STOP HEADACHES

1 lemon, peeled

4 lettuce leaves

2 spinach leaves

1 bunch purple grapes

3 carrots

½-inch slice ginger root

14 HELPS PREVENT HEART DISEASE

2 oranges *or* tangerines, peeled

1 lemon, peeled

2 stalks celery, leaves removed

2 tomatoes

1 red radish

¼ red onion

1 clove garlic (*optional*)

15 CAN HELP LOWER CHOLESTEROL

1 orange *or* tangerine, with some peel

1 grapefruit, peeled

1 tomato

1 clove garlic *or* ¼ red onion

2 dandelion leaves *or* 2 cabbage leaves

1 red radish and tops

16 CAN HELP PREVENT OR LOWER HIGH BLOOD PRESSURE

2 oranges, peeled

2-inch slice of watermelon

2 stalks celery, leaves removed

½ cup chopped parsley

½ cup chopped fennel

4 lettuce leaves

17 CAN HELP CALM AN IRRITABLE OR INFLAMED BOWEL

1 orange, peeled

½ carrot

2 green apples, peeled

½-inch slice ginger root

3 stalks celery

1 handful fresh mixed herbs, chopped—mint, parsley, basil, cilantro

Add ⅛ cup aloe vera juice

Aloe juice should be purchased, or prepared with care; the outer leaf is a strong laxative

18 OF PARTICULAR HELP IN CLEANSING AND HEALING THE LIVER

1 lemon, with some peel

2 red apples

½ carrot

2 dandelion leaves *or* 2 cabbage leaves

½ cup broccoli florets

1 clove garlic *or* ¼ red onion

1 cup fresh mixed herbs, chopped—parsley, mint, cilantro, basil, chives

This is a strong mixture and may be diluted with 1 cup water *or* dandelion root tea

19 OF PARTICULAR HELP IN REMOVING FAT FROM THE LIVER

1 lemon *or* grapefruit, peeled

2 carrots

1 clove garlic *or* ¼ red onion

½-inch round fennel

¼ beetroot

2 dandelion leaves *or* 2 cabbage leaves

1 apple may be added for taste

20 GOOD FOR THE GALLBLADDER AND BILIARY TRACT

1 lemon, with some peel

2 fresh dandelion leaves *or* cabbage leaves

¼ beetroot

1 medium apple

2 Brussels sprouts

1 large tomato

21 GOOD FOR PEOPLE WITH LIVER INFLAMMATION (HEPATITIS)

1 orange, peeled

1 lemon, peeled

2 carrots

1 apple, with skin

1 to 2 cloves garlic *or* ¼ red onion

½ beetroot and tops

½ cup watercress

1 handful fresh herbs, chopped—lemon thyme, mint, oregano

22 HELPS PREVENT MACULAR DEGENERATION

1 orange *or* mandarin, with some peel

½ lemon, peeled

1 blood orange *or* grapefruit, peeled

2 carrots

1 tomato

¼ beetroot and tops

2 spinach leaves

½ glove garlic (*optional*)

23 HELPS PREVENT HOT FLASHES

2 oranges, peeled but with pith

½ cup alfalfa *or* bean sprouts

2 lettuce leaves

2-inch slice watermelon

1 small cucumber, peeled

¼ beetroot

1 handful fresh herbs, chopped—sage, mint, parsley

24 CAN HELP DELAY OR PREVENT OSTEOPOROSIS

2 oranges, peeled

6 spinach leaves

4 string beans, chopped

½ cup alfalfa *or* bean sprouts

1 apple

25 REDUCES PREMENSTRUAL PAIN AND REDUCES HEAVY BLEEDING

2 oranges, peeled but with pith

3 spinach leaves, chopped

¼ beetroot and tops

2 lettuce leaves

½ cup chopped parsley

1 apple

26 REDUCES MENSTRUAL PAIN

1 orange, with some peel and pith left on

½ cup raspberries

2 spinach leaves

2 carrots

¼ beetroot

½-inch slice ginger root

1 Tbsp. of flaxseed oil

27 GOOD FOR PEOPLE WITH SINUS PROBLEMS AND HAY FEVER

1 orange, peeled

1 lemon, peeled

3 small red radishes

½-inch ginger root

1 clove garlic, *or* ¼ red onion, *or* ½-inch slice horseradish

2-inch slice fresh pineapple

1 carrot

This juice will be spicy; if necessary, dilute with water, *or* apple juice, *or* cold herbal tea

28 HELPS PREVENT AND REDUCE ACNE

1 orange, peeled but with pith left on

1 lemon, peeled

2 carrots

½ beetroot and tops

2 stalks celery, leaves removed

1 handful mixed fresh herbs, chopped—basil, mint, lemon thyme

29 HELPS CLEANSE THE SKIN AND REDUCE RASHES

2 oranges, peeled but with pith

1 cup strawberries

1 handful fresh mixed herbs, chopped—mint, cilantro, parsley, basil

1 tsp. of honey and crushed ice, if desired

30 A POWERFUL ANTIOXIDANT

1 orange, with peel

1 lemon, peeled

1 pomegranate, its seeds and flesh

2-inch slice fresh pineapple

2 apricots, pitted

1 cup pureed blueberries

31 CALMS THE STOMACH AND HELPS PREVENT ULCERS

1 lime, peeled

2 large cabbage leaves, chopped

1 apple, peeled

1 papaya, without seeds

1 pear

1 handful fresh mixed herbs, chopped—mint, cilantro,
   parsley, basil

32 GOOD FOR PEOPLE WITH THYROID PROBLEMS

1 orange, peeled

1 red radish

2 carrots

¼ beetroot and tops

2 lettuce leaves

½-inch ginger root

1 tsp. kelp powder (*optional*)

33 CAN HELP BOOST A SLUGGISH METABOLISM AND INCREASE WEIGHT LOSS

1 orange, peeled

1 grapefruit, peeled

1 carrot

2 stalks celery, leaves removed

½-inch slice ginger root

2 radishes

Pinch cayenne

Dilute by half with strong green tea

34 POWERFUL LIVER CLEANSER

1 grapefruit, peeled but with pith

½ cup green string beans

3 broccoli florets

2 Brussels sprouts

1 carrot

Dilute by half with water

35 REDUCES CELLULITE

1 orange, with some peel

1 lemon, peeled

1 apple, with skin

1 plum, with skin

1 handful fresh mixed herbs, chopped—mint, cilantro,
   parsley, basil

2 stalks celery, leaves removed

36 HELPS TO BURN FAT

1 orange, with some peel

1 grapefruit, with pith

2 handfuls fresh mixed herbs, chopped—mint, cilantro,
   parsley, basil

1 radish

1 apple, peeled

¼ beetroot

1 spring onion

37 GOOD ALL-AROUND CLEANSING JUICE FOR WEIGHT LOSS AND ENERGY BOOST

½ grapefruit, peeled

1 red apple

1 dandelion leaf *or* 1 broccoli floret

1 tomato

1 nectarine (stone removed)

2-inch slice red onion

2 Brussels sprouts

2 beet leaves

38 GOOD ALL-AROUND JUICE FOR INCREASING ENERGY

2 oranges, peeled

¼ cantaloupe

½ cup bean sprouts (alfalfa *or* snow peas)

1 dandelion leaf *or* 1 broccoli floret

1 spinach leaf

1 carrot

39 GOOD ALL-AROUND CLEANSER TO REDUCE ACIDITY
IN THE BODY

½ grapefruit, peeled

1 lemon, peeled

2 stalks celery, leaves removed

1 cucumber

1 red radish

2-inch slice fresh pineapple

½-inch ginger root

40 GOOD ALL-AROUND JUICE FOR BOOSTING ENERGY

1 orange, peeled

1 lemon, peeled

4 spinach leaves

2 carrots

4 string beans, chopped

1 peach, peeled (stone removed)

41 HELPS FIGHT ALLERGIES AND HAY FEVER

1 red radish

1 clove garlic *or* ½ red onion

1 carrot

1 pear

2 cabbage leaves

1 orange, peeled

42 BOOSTS THE LIVER AND IMMUNE SYSTEM, AND
REDUCES HEAVY METALS

1 lemon, peeled

½-inch fresh ginger root

1 apple

1 carrot

2 dandelion leaves *or* 2 cabbage leaves

2 handfuls fresh mixed herbs, chopped—mint, cilantro,
parsley, basil

¼ red onion

43 ACTS AS AN ANTIBIOTIC AND ANTISEPTIC FOR ALL
INFECTIONS, ELIMINATES PARASITES

1 carrot

½ beetroot, including some green tops

2 spinach leaves

2 apples, with skin

½-inch fresh ginger root

½-inch horseradish root

1 clove garlic (*optional*) *or* ½ red onion

½ cup watercress (*optional*)

May want to dilute with water

44 HELPS REDUCE INFLAMMATION IN THE JOINTS

4 stalks celery

1 carrot

2 medium apples, cored, with skin

7 oz. fresh alfalfa sprouts

1 small handful of grapes

½ to 1 clove garlic (*optional*) *or* ¼ red onion

½-inch ginger root

1 handful fresh mixed herbs, chopped—mint, cilantro,
parsley, basil

45 HELPS REDUCE SYMPTOMS OF ASTHMA

1 carrot

1 orange *or* ½ grapefruit, leave some pith on

1 green apple, peel left on

1 pear, peeled

¼-inch fresh ginger root

1 clove garlic *or* ¼ red onion

2 cabbage leaves

4-inch slice fresh pineapple

46 HELPS PREVENT OR REDUCE HIGH BLOOD PRESSURE

3 stalks celery

½ cucumber, peeled

½ cup chopped fennel

1 spring onion *or* 1 clove garlic

1 apple

1 handful fresh mixed herbs, chopped—mint, cilantro, parsley, basil

1 orange *or* ½ grapefruit

47 PROVIDES ENERGY BOOST FOR PEOPLE WITH CHRONIC FATIGUE SYNDROME

1 carrot

½ medium beetroot with top leaves

2 turnip leaves

1 cup fresh parsley, chopped

2 spinach leaves *or* 2 cabbage leaves

1 medium apple, cored, with skin

½ clove garlic

1 peach *or* nectarine (stone removed)

⅓ cup wheatgrass, if available

48 HELPS RELIEVE CONSTIPATION

2 spinach, dandelion, *or* cabbage leaves

1 green apple, with skin

4 oz. dried prunes, pits removed

4 oz. figs, fresh if possible, otherwise dried

2 oz. of fresh rhubarb (red stalk only)

2 oz. fresh cherries (*optional*), pits removed

Soak dried fruit in water overnight so they are soft
enough to pass through the juicer

49 GOOD FOR THE URINARY TRACT AND REDUCES
CYSTITIS AND INFECTIONS

½ cup fresh cranberries, if available

2 stalks celery, leaves removed

1 medium green apple, with skin

½ grapefruit

½ clove garlic *or* ¼ red onion

1 small cucumber, peeled

1 medium carrot

1 red radish and top leaves

50 GOOD FOR HEARTBURN AND GASTROESOPHAGEAL
REFLUX

1 large red apple, with skin, *or* 1 large pear, with skin

2 stalks celery

1 cup fresh alfalfa sprouts

1 medium carrot

1 or 2 large cabbage leaves

1 handful seeded black cherries

51 GOOD FOR STOMACH INFECTIONS

¼ pineapple, peeled

½ cup chopped cauliflower with stem and leaf

½ cup watercress

2 cabbage leaves

1 red radish with top leaves

½ to 1 clove garlic (*optional*)

1 pomegranate (when in season), its seeds and flesh

52 GOOD FOR REDUCING GAS AND STOMACH BLOATING

1 cabbage leaf

½-inch fresh ginger root

3-inch slice fresh pineapple

½ cup mint leaves, chopped

1 green apple, peeled

53 REDUCES THE SYMPTOMS OF ENDOMETRIOSIS AND
PROMOTES HORMONAL BALANCE

1 carrot

1 cabbage leaf

1-inch fresh ginger root

½ cup coriander leaves, chopped

¼ pineapple (remove skin and rough, dry pieces)

1 whole orange *or* grapefruit, peeled

3 very dark green spinach leaves

¼ cup parsley, chopped

54 CAN HELP PREVENT HAIR LOSS

1 cup alfalfa sprouts

2 cabbage leaves *or* 2 Brussels sprouts

1 medium carrot

1 red apple

1-inch slice red onion

1 medium beetroot and tops

½ to 1 clove garlic (*optional*)

2 medium slices watermelon (to sweeten, if desired)

55 HELPS RELIEVE OR PREVENT INSOMNIA

2 to 3 large outer leaves of lettuce

1 whole pear *or* apple, peeled

1 carrot

1 sweet potato, peeled and chopped

½ medium bulb of fennel, chopped

1 grapefruit

56 HELPS PREVENT OR RELIEVE THE SYMPTOMS OF JET LAG

1 grapefruit, peeled

½ medium pineapple, peeled, cored, and chopped

½-inch fresh ginger root

1 handful fresh mixed herbs, chopped—mint, cilantro, parsley, basil

57 HELPS KEEP KIDNEYS HEALTHY AND REDUCES KIDNEY STONES

5-inch slice watermelon

1 small cucumber, peeled

1 peach (stone removed)

1 cup parsley, chopped

4 string beans, chopped

1 spring onion

58 HELPS PREVENT CHRONIC INFECTION/ INFLAMMATION OF THE GUMS (PERIODONTAL DISEASE) AND FRESHENS THE BREATH

2 to 3 dandelion leaves *or* spinach leaves

3 handfuls fresh mixed herbs, chopped—mint, cilantro, parsley, basil, thyme, oregano

½-inch fresh ginger root

1 whole apple
1 whole orange *or* grapefruit
1 lemon
1 carrot

59 ANTIAGING JUICE
5 oz. blueberries *or* blackberries
5 oz. raspberries
½-inch fresh ginger root
½ clove garlic *or* ¼ red onion
1 grapefruit with white pith
1 orange, pith on

Variety: Good *for* You!

I'd say it should be obvious by now that there are almost as many different fruit, vegetable, and fresh herb juicing combinations as there are moons in our galaxy. The 60 or so recipes I've listed here contain only a fraction of the fruits and vegetables that are available—at least seasonally—for juicing. And the only things that will limit the number of juice combinations you can enjoy during a fast are your imagination and your taste buds.

Speaking of taste buds, if you are like me and enjoy an occasional dessert...well, there is no reason to deprive yourself just because you happen to be fasting. One of my personal favorites is a "Berry Delicious" smoothie, which is made with 4 ounces of strawberries, 4 ounces of blueberries, and 4 ounces of raspberries. If you want it sweeter, just add some stevia, which is a naturally sweet herb. Toss the berries into a blender with a handful of ice and blend away. Mmmm, good!

For another nice dessert treat, try:

2 bunches of grapes, white or dark

2 lemons, peeled and juiced

¼ cup fresh mint, chopped

1 pint (16 oz.) water

1 tsp. honey or stevia, to taste

Wash the grapes and process them in your juicer, and then add lemon juice, chopped mint, water, and honey and serve over crushed ice.

Delicious!

As you experiment on your own with various juice combinations and experience the "healthy joy" they'll bring to your life, just remember three things:

- Use organically grown fruits, vegetables, and herbs whenever possible.
- The fresher your fruits and vegetables, the tastier they'll be and the higher their nutrient content— so try to use produce that is in season and (even better) produce that is locally grown.
- If a juice combination tastes good to you, drink it (then note it in this book or in a journal of your favorite recipes). If it doesn't, experiment with some extra apple, watermelon, or pear until it is acceptable.

Now, quit reading for a while and enjoy a glass of fresh, healthy, and delicious juices. It will definitely add to the quality of your day—and that's true, regardless of whether at this particular moment you are fasting or not!

8

Ending Your Fast Properly

I truly hope that you will find your first fast to be an uplifting and enjoyable experience that you may even not want to end. One of the most common reactions to juice fasting is a feeling of physical and mental "lightness" that comes by replacing heavy, processed, cooked, and sugared foods with lighter, more refreshing juices made from fruits, herbs, and vegetables.

It turns out that, for some of you at least, the longer you go without following a traditional diet, the less you will miss it. With all fasters, though, whether juice or otherwise, the day comes when good health requires that they break their fast and resume a "normal" diet. (More on that "normal" diet toward the end of this chapter.)

I can list a variety of reasons why you might choose to end your fast. These can range from reaching your predetermined fasting goal, to needing to take a business trip, to leaving on vacation with the family. Often, people just listen to their bodies and end their fast when a strong desire for food returns. This desire can manifest itself in myriad ways. It might be that you constantly dream about eating, or you could experience an almost uncontrollable urge to search the trunk of your car for the package of peanuts you seem to remember seeing there. Maybe you've become obsessed with what your coworkers will be eating for lunch, or you envy your dog for having a big hambone to chew on.

Regardless of the specifics, if your body (or your mind) is telling you that it's time to end your fast, then listen. It knows what it's talking about. A growing sense of hunger or a sense of urgency about the need to eat—especially if you've been fasting for a week or more—are signs that your body is crying out for something it's not getting.

But again, remember that everyone is different, which makes it rather difficult to make a "one scenario fits all" recommendation about the right time to break a fast. All I can say, with any real certainty, is that if you pay attention to what your body is trying to tell you, it's almost impossible to go wrong.

Once you do make a decision to break your fast, you may be surprised how difficult it can be to actually stop, particularly for longer fasts. Some say it's even harder than the fast itself—in part because, consciously or unconsciously, your mind and your body are reaping some pretty powerful health benefits that they really don't want to give up. And then there is always the decision of "What should I eat first?"

Learn How NOT to Break Your Fast

I have heard anecdotal stories of people breaking a fast by eating a 16-ounce steak with all the trimmings, or perhaps a large pizza or something equally hearty, and washing it all down with quart of soda or a pitcher of beer. I say "anecdotal" because I personally have never met anyone so foolish as to end a fast in this manner, though I can't swear that it hasn't been tried. I would be willing to bet, however, that if you were to break your fast by eating a steak and drinking a large quantity of beer...well, it wouldn't happen more than once.

It would be, to say the least, a discomforting experience. And most of that experience would likely be spent grasping your stomach and moaning and groaning in near proximity to a bathroom.

I'd compare ending a fast with a pizza to going to the beach in midsummer and lying out all day under a hot sun. If eating the pizza (lying in the sun) is something you have been doing all along—if it's something your body is used to—then, leaving aside the possibility of skin cancer, it is not that big of a deal. Your stomach will gladly accept the pizza (or, as the case may be, your skin will just get a little darker).

But, on the other hand, if you are pale as a ghost and haven't seen the sun in weeks, and then decide to spend a full day at the beach, sans sunscreen, you are going to fry like the proverbial egg on a hot sidewalk. And you'll be miserable for days as a result.

My point here: Ease in to breaking a fast, particularly if it lasts longer than 48 hours. A good rule of thumb is that you should take half as long to resume your prefast eating habits as the time spent fasting. Some experienced fasters will recommend that you take more time; I doubt anyone would suggest less. But I believe that if you juice fast for, say, seven days, then taking somewhere between three and four days to ease back into your regular eating patterns will be sufficient.

Ease Out of Your Fast

Here's how to end your fast and get back to your regular patterns. Your first meal following a fast should always consist of fresh, nonspicy, bland foods such as fresh fruits, herbs, and vegetables; fresh tomato soup; or perhaps a bowl of freshly made vegetable soup with a fewer than usual number of vegetables and a watered-down broth; you may have sea salt and pepper to season, if desired. Whatever you choose to eat, have a small portion. eat it slowly, and chew the food well.

Not overeating is important—it's super important. Now, you might be thinking that this is true in every situation involving food, and you'd be correct. It is particularly crucial, however, when you're reintroducing your stomach to food following a fast. Your body's tendency to keep your portions small at that time will be a normal physiological response to fasting: After more than a day with no food, your stomach will start shrinking and gradually lose its ability to hold the quantities you may have formerly eaten.

You'll want to stick with the same diet on the first and second days after a fast, though you might add a cup of natural plain yogurt or a small portion of raw nuts, and even a boiled or baked potato (without toppings). You still will need to stay away from sugar and preservatives, though by the third day you can add a piece of whole-grain bread with natural butter or hummus and a slice of avocado. You'll find your appetite gradually growing as your stomach starts to expand and gets used to again receiving food, but try to restrain yourself this third day and stick with only the healthiest of foods. Burgers and fries aren't going anywhere; they will still be around in another few days, but I sincerely hope that you won't be eating them regularly, anyway!

You can add more and different foods on each day succeeding a lengthy fast. Just remember to drink at least 48 ounces of water each day (six 8-ounce glasses), and don't forget that you can always fall back on those delicious smoothies made with fresh fruits.

Over the years, I've found years that citrus fruits, particularly oranges, are a great favorite for breaking a fast, as are watermelon, apples, pears, and peaches, along with fresh, sweet berries and grapes. So many of the fruits that tasted so good as juices will now taste just as yummy to you as solid foods. And they'll still offer the same healthy and body-enriching ingredients. Another favorite among many people are dried fruits, which can be soaked overnight in water to make them easy to chew and digest.

I think you'll find that breaking a fast can be turned into both an easy and pleasurable experience, as long as you take it slow and avoid sugar-laden, rich, highly processed, and deep-fried foods.

Use your common sense and avoid foods that will upset a stomach that's used to being empty.

Consider Ways to Improve Your Normal Diet

At this point, I'd also like to recommend that you end your fast—whether it's your first fast or your tenth—with a plan to gradually change your overall eating habits for the better. Now, there's nothing wrong about wanting, or having, an *occasional* grilled-cheese sandwich, or an order of deep-fried onion rings, or a hot-fudge sundae, or a piece of chocolate cake. For many people, that's the "normal" diet I mentioned earlier.

We all have our favorite foods—foods that often aren't the healthiest items on the menu—and I see no problem with your indulging yourself from time to time...say, four or six times a month. (That's single incidents, not days!)

But you must remember that up to 80 percent of the toxins in your body will come from the foods you eat. Therefore, juice fasting and the detoxification process it sets in motion won't be nearly as effective in the long term if you continue to dump large amounts of old or new toxins into your body in between fasts.

This doesn't mean that you can never again enjoy the foods you've come to love. As I've just said, you simply enjoy them less often. And when you do 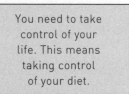 make up your mind to start changing your diet for the better, I can guarantee that you'll start feeling better. A juice fast can give you the first and exciting taste of a new, healthier life full of energy. If you are like many of my patients, that first taste can be addictive! It can lead to an eventual and beneficial 180-degree turn around. Whereas you once were eating processed and sugar-laden foods that added toxicity to your body, you may find yourself switching to fresh fruits, vegetables, fresh herbs, legumes, raw nuts and seeds, and lean organic meats that are largely free of additives, preservatives, and harmful chemicals.

As more than one writer on healthy eating has noted, your body is your friend and it only wants what is best for you. It wants to be healthy. It wants to help you live a long and satisfying life. But those goals can only be achieved if you do your part by adopting a healthier diet. The bottom line here: Take care of your body and it, in turn, will take care of you.

Finally, I must stress that juice fasting—despite its many wonders and benefits—is not intended to take the place of professional medical care. It should not be considered a miracle cure for disease, nor is it a replacement for surgery or any other type of medical procedure. Instead, what fasting with raw fruit, raw vegetable, and fresh herb juices does for most people is make them healthier and less prone to diseases.

> You need to take control of your life. This means taking control of your diet.

Enjoy the Health Benefits of Regular Juice Fasting

To recap some of the benefits of juice fasting, as discussed in previous chapters, it will enable you to:

- Fight off diseases, especially infections and chronic inflammation, which lead to degenerative diseases
- Heal faster from existing illnesses
- Reduce the load of parasites in your bowel
- Reduce your body's total load of toxic chemicals and heavy metals
- Reduce intestinal diseases such as inflamed bowel pockets (diverticulitis), inflammatory bowel diseases, and constipation
- Improve the function of your kidneys
- Reduce gallstones and gall bladder diseases
- Improve liver function
- Repair liver damage, including "fatty liver"
- Reduce arthritis and fibromyalgia
- Reduce headaches, even migraines
- Control your weight more easily
- Boost a sluggish metabolism
- Reduce cellulite
- Reduce your risk of cancer by a significant amount
- Reduce your risk of Alzheimer's dementia
- Be sharper mentally and have more-balanced moods
- Be more physically active and energetic
- Live a longer, more enjoyable, more productive life
- Slow down the aging process
- Know that you are being a good friend to your own body and are in more control of your life

As you have undoubtedly figured out by now, I am a tremendous believer in the powerful and life-changing benefits of juice fasting. If I weren't, I would not use it in my own life as well as in my medical practice. Aside from juice fasting, if more people did raw juicing regularly, we would see enormous preventative health benefits in the world's population.

At the extremes of age, in the very young and the very old, raw juicing can strengthen our greatest health asset—our immune system. If pregnant women juiced regularly, we would see fewer congenital abnormalities and less cancer in their offspring. If busy and stressed executives would organize their administrative assistants to prepare raw fruit, vegetable, and herbal juices instead of sugar-laden coffee and donuts, we would see fewer nervous breakdowns and less alcoholism. If breast-feeding mothers would juice daily, we would see less postpartum depression. If those prone to headaches who depend on taking painkillers would juice regularly, they would achieve a much higher quality of life. If those with chronic infections, whether viral or bacterial, would use my juice recipes regularly, we would see less use of antibiotic drugs and less antibiotic resistance in microorganisms. Although I can give no promises, I have seen raw juicing cure cancer, resolve several different types of liver disease, and overcome chronic fatigue syndrome. Never underestimate the power of raw juicing!

I am pleased to have had this opportunity to share with you the healthy and healing properties of something so simple, so affordable, and so easily obtainable as a glass of fresh raw vegetable, fruit, and herb juices.

Juice fasting is not only a key to a better life, it's a key to life itself. *Drink up!*

Testimonials to the Power of Raw Juicing

Raw juicing truly needs to become a part of your lifestyle. For me and many of my patients, it has become an essential part of life. Here are a few testimonials about raw juicing that show its power.

Migraine Headaches

Mary had suffered with frequent and severe migraines. She had been taking powerful analgesics for years, because the preventative drugs had caused unacceptable side effects and were not very effective. I recommended that Mary drink two large glasses daily of juice freshly made from citrus fruits, carrots, apples, cabbage, and fresh green herbs. I also told her to take a magnesium supplement in a dose of 400 mg. daily. Mary was desperate, because her life had become very miserable and the analgesics were making her extremely tired.

After six weeks of juicing, Mary was amazed by the improvement in her health and found that the headaches were much less frequent. After six months of juicing she told me that she rarely got headaches and if she did they were small, petty ones that did not last. Mary found that if she did wake with a headache the raw juice would relieve it within half an hour.

Bowel Cancer

Graham was a 46-year-old merchant banker who had lived a high-pressured life and had not had much time to look after his health. One day he was shocked to see blood in his bowel movements, so he went to a bowel specialist who did extensive tests. The results were not good: The doctor had found a large cancer in Graham's large bowel (colon). Graham was urged to have surgery and radiation therapy to eradicate the tumor. Although the tumor was large, it was not producing any symptoms such as pain or obstruction, so Graham did not have to panic.

He went to see a naturopath, who recommended that he try natural therapies first. In cases of cancer, such decisions are extremely difficult, but in Graham's case he was categorical that he did not want to try invasive or destructive treatment, and he also understood that his cancer was a result of his poor diet and lifestyle.

Graham drastically changed his lifestyle and began a program of juicing whereby he drank about two quarts of raw juice everyday. He chose many types of vegetables, fruits, and fresh green herbs. He used a powerful juicer that had a grinding action, which enabled him to extract the maximum amount of juice from the produce and did not overheat the produce while it was being processed into juice. After six months of this juicing program, there was no sign of any cancer in his bowel and he felt energetic and well. Of course, the surgeon was not pleased, but was at least reassured by the fact that Graham had agreed to have regular colonoscopies to make sure the cancer did not reappear.

I firmly believe that raw juicing is an essential part of any treatment plan for cancer patients, and that regular juicing will also greatly reduce the risk of cancer developing.

Cystitis

Belinda was a 56-year-old woman who had come to see me for a chronic and painful condition called interstitial cystitis. In this condition the whole thickness of the bladder wall is inflamed, causing symptoms such as suprapubic pain, urinary frequency and urgency, painful intercourse, and burning while passing urine. Belinda had tried the usual gamut of conventional treatments, such as laser therapy to the mucosal lining of the bladder and repeated courses of antibiotic drugs. These treatments produced only short-lived benefit and had side effects, and over the years her bladder inflammation had become much worse.

I started Belinda on a course of nutritional supplements, including the minerals selenium and magnesium. I assured her that if she became a fan of raw juicing she could beat this terrible disease. Obviously, she was desperate, as many folks are, when they finally come to the last resort—if only they had found out about juicing earlier!

I told Belinda to make juice from citrus fruits, celery, cucumber, zucchini, carrot, beets, red radish, red onion, and apples. After three months of juicing, Belinda was symptom free and became one of my biggest supporters.

Lung Disease

Sophie came to see me in a pathetic state of health. Although she was only 56 years old, she looked literally like "a fish out of water" as she sat before me with blue-colored lips, rapid breathing, an audible wheeze, and a congestive, rattly cough. She was married to a wealthy businessman and life should have been good for her, and yet she lived a life of physical torture.

Sophie's symptoms were due to a severe lung disease known as chronic obstructive airways disease. She also had bronchiectasis, a condition in which the bronchial tubes are swollen and full of infected mucus. These lung diseases kept her in a permanent state of oxygen deprivation and fatigue. Sophie no longer responded to antibiotics, as the common bacteria that colonized her lungs were all resistant to these drugs after many years of repeated courses.

I started Sophie on a program of physiotherapy and nutritional supplements, including selenium, zinc, fish oil, and vitamin C. I believed that the most important thing for her—and, indeed, it was a matter of life or death—was to strengthen both her immune system and her lungs. To achieve this end, I explained to her the pivotal role of raw juicing. Sophie was lucky enough to have a full-time housekeeper, as she would not have had the energy to make the juices herself. Six weeks after starting her raw-juice regimen, Sophie returned to see me. She had a much better color and the deathly blue cyanosis previously seen in her lips had gone. She was breathing much more easily, and her cough no longer stopped her from sleeping.

Today Sophie lives a relatively normal life. She still has permanent lung damage, but it does not prevent her from functioning. I am sure that raw juicing has added many years of enjoyable life for this poor woman.

It is a pity that children with chronic lung diseases, such as cystic fibrosis and severe asthma, are not provided with the benefits of raw juicing simply because their families are ignorant of the healing power it provides.

Other Books from Ulysses Press

COMPLETE COLON CLEANSE: THE AT-HOME DETOX PROGRAM
TO RESTORE GOOD HEALTH, BOOST VITALITY, AND ENSURE
LONGEVITY
Dr. Edward Group, $12.95
Packed with info on powerful, all-natural cleanses as well as
advice on long-term colon health, this book is the ultimate tool
for relieving colon-related illnesses, restoring vitality, and obtain-
ing maximum colon health.

THE COMPLETE MASTER CLEANSE: A STEP-BY-STEP GUIDE TO
MAXIMIZING THE BENEFITS OF THE LEMONADE DIET
Tom Woloshyn, $11.95
Fasting for days while drinking a lemonade-like blend of clear
spring water, cayenne pepper and citrus juice has proven to be a
safe, simple and yet powerful way to cleanse the body of toxins.
This book goes beyond basic information on how to do the
cleanse—which can be learned in minutes—by guiding readers
step by step through the entire cleansing process.

THE EASY GL DIET HANDBOOK: LOSE WEIGHT WITH THE
REVOLUTIONARY GLYCEMIC LOAD PROGRAM
Dr. Fedon Alexander Lindberg, $10.00
Using these more accurate and sensible GL scores, *The Easy GL
Diet Handbook* offers a plan for healthy weight loss and reduced
risk of diabetes that's easier to follow. It also includes numerous
foods that the Atkins, South Beach, and GI diets wrongly con-
sider "off-limits."

THE GL COOKBOOK AND DIET PLAN: A GLYCEMIC LOAD
WEIGHT-LOSS PROGRAM WITH OVER 150 DELICIOUS RECIPES
Nigel Denby, $12.95
Offers a vast selection of GL-scored recipes so dieters can choose
dishes they love while following a proven program for permanent
weight loss without hunger.

THE LEPTIN BOOST DIET: UNLEASH YOUR FAT-CONTROLLING HORMONES FOR MAXIMUM WEIGHT LOSS

Scott Isaacs, M.D., $14.95

A series of recent medical breakthroughs have confirmed what physicians suspected all along—obesity is a hormonal disorder. *The Leptin Boost Diet* transforms these findings into a unique and easy-to-follow weight-loss program that is perfect for people whose out-of-balance hormones make it impossible to lose weight on other diets.

THE LIVER AND GALLBLADDER MIRACLE CLEANSE: AN ALL-NATURAL, AT-HOME FLUSH TO PURIFY AND REJUVENATE YOUR BODY

Andreas Moritz, $14.95

Illustrates how to recognize stone buildup and provides do-it-yourself instructions for painlessly flushing them out of the body.

THE PH BALANCE DIET: RESTORE YOUR ACID-ALKALINE LEVELS TO ELIMINATE TOXINS AND LOSE WEIGHT

Bharti Vyas & Suzanne Le Quesne, $12.95

Tells how to pH-test one's body, correct imbalances, and eliminate toxic overload by following a dietary way of life that works. An easy-to-follow section with over 40 recipes is included to help guide readers through the plan.

To order these books call 800-377-2542 or 510-601-8301, fax 510-601-8307, e-mail ulysses@ulyssespress.com, or write to Ulysses Press, P.O. Box 3440, Berkeley, CA 94703. All retail orders are shipped free of charge. California residents must include sales tax. Allow two to three weeks for delivery.

About the Author

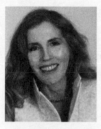**Sandra Cabot, M.D.**, is the medical and executive director of the Australian National Health Advisory Service, which publishes her books and helps to raise money for women refugees and firefighters in New South Wales, Australia.

She graduated with honors in medicine and surgery from the University of Adelaide in South Australia in 1975. As part of her extracurricular medical training, she studied naturopathic medicine, because at a young age she could see beyond the limitations of drug-oriented medicine, which treated symptoms and not the causes of disease.

Dr. Cabot began her medical career in 1980 as a general practitioner obstetrician-gynecologist, practicing in Sydney, Australia. During the mid-1980s she spent six months working as a volunteer doctor at the Leyman Hospital, then the largest missionary hospital in northern India.

Dr. Cabot has written several ground-breaking books on hormones, cleansing diets, weight loss, cholesterol, diabetes, and detoxing, among other subjects. Her *Liver Cleansing Diet* has sold over two million copies worldwide, has been translated into six languages (including Arabic), and was awarded the prestigious Australian People's Choice Award for the most popular nonfiction book in 1996.

Dr. Cabot is also an experienced commercial pilot and flies herself to seminars throughout Australia, often visiting remote areas. She does regular work for the Angel Flight Charity, which provides free transport for patients with chronic and severe disabilities in remote areas of her country.

She has conducted health seminars all over the world and is frequently asked to lecture for numerous health organizations, such as the American Liver Foundation and the Annual Hepatitis Symposium. She maintains an active medical practice and does research into liver diseases.

Dr. Cabot may be contacted at P.O. Box 5070, Glendale, Arizona 85312; telephone (623) 334-3232. Visit her websites www.liverdoctor.com and www.weightcontroldoctor.com.